Children Without Childhood

Children Without Childhood

A Study of Childhood Schizophrenia

BENJAMIN B. WOLMAN

*Professor, Doctoral Program in
Clinical Psychology, Long Island University;
Dean, Institute of Applied Psychoanalysis*

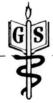

GRUNE & STRATTON New York and London

Library of Congress Catalog Card Number 71-100072

Printed in U. S. A.
(PC-B)

To children
whose childhood was taken away . . .

Acknowledgments

The author and the publisher gratefully acknowledge the permission to quote from:

Gesell, A., and Amatruda, C.S. *Developmental diagnosis: Normal and abnormal child development: Clinical methods and pediatric applications* (2nd ed.). New York: Hoeber Medical Division, Harper & Row, 1947, p. 327.

Goldfarb, W. *Childhood schizophrenia.* Cambridge: Harvard University Press, 1961.

Halpern, Florence. Diagnostic methods in childhood disorders. In B.B. Wolman (Ed.). *Handbook of clinical psychology.* New York: McGraw-Hill, 1965, pp. 628-634.

Kallman, F.J. The genetic theory of schizophrenia. *American Journal of Psychiatry,* 1964, *103,* 316.

Kringlen, E. Schizophrenia in twins: An epidemiological clinical study. *Psychiatry,* 1966, *29,* 172-184.

Spitz, R.A. Hospitalism: A follow-up report on investigations described in Vol. I, 1945. *The Psychoanalytic Study of the Child,* 1946, *2,* 113-117.

Wolman, B.B. Mental health and mental disorders. In B.B. Wolman (Ed.). *Handbook of clinical psychology.* New York: McGraw-Hill, 1965, pp. 992-993.

Wolman, B.B. *Vectoriasis praecox or the group of schizophrenias.* Springfield, Illinois: Charles C Thomas, 1966, pp. 79-83.

Miss Susan Knapp, doctoral candidate in clinical psychology at Long Island University, offered invaluable aid in preparation of the manuscript. In the last stage of work, I was assisted by Kathryn Bevacqua, Barbara Dobrin, Sondra Gerber, and Stuart Sparber.

B.B.W.

Preface

In the thirties, I worked in an institution for abnormal children overseas, where we had eighty to ninety children at age levels of five through eighteen. It was at that time that I became puzzled by the peculiar background of the children; whenever a child was schizophrenic, his parents inadvertently hated one another and used the child emotionally.

In the late thirties and in the forties, I was director of a children's clinic and institution for disturbed children, in Israel. There I became more and more acquainted with the uneven mental performance and bizarre behavior of schizophrenic and preschizophrenic children. I worked closely with the parents of these children, and the peculiar intrafamilial interaction became more and more apparent. Whether the parents came from Europe, Africa, or Asia, whether they were Jewish, Moslem, or Christian, the pattern was always the same.

During World War Two, I was in charge of educational services for families of soldiers in Israel. I coordinated sociotherapeutic programs for families separated by war, and I had the chance to study broken and not-yet-broken homes. Again, I found the same peculiar intrafamilial interaction in families who had a schizophrenic child.

The idea of formalizing my findings developed gradually. While working with men and officers in the Israeli War of Independence, it occurred to me that the morale in the Israeli Army was based on different factors than those described by American psychologists. It was certainly neither J. L. Moreno's acceptance-rejection or popularity issue, nor K. Lewin's field theory. It was the *goal,* the idea, that captivated the minds of Israeli boys and girls and turned practically every Israeli private into a hero.

A study in classroom relationship started earlier and published in Hebrew (1949) led to two formal concepts: power and acceptance. Power was defined as the ability to satisfy needs, the ultimate need being survival. Acceptance was defined as the willingness to do or not to do so. Children in classrooms willingly obeyed teachers perceived as strong (able to satisfy needs) and friendly (willing to do so); in that study distinct levels in peer relationship have been delineated.

A further classification of the interactional patterns was developed in several theoretical and experimental studies (some of them included in the bibliography at the end of this volume). Most of these experiments were conducted in the fifties in this country. Three types of relationships have been distinguished. An *instrumental* relationship is the infant-mother relationship, where the infant *receives* all the support and his survival depends upon these supplies. A *mutual* (or mutual acceptance) relationship is practiced in sex and marriage, whenever each party intends to receive satisfaction and aims at the same time at the gratification of the needs of the other party. A *vectorial* relationship is the mother-infant relationship, where mother is willing to give everything away for the child's survival without asking anything in return.

A normal individual acts in an instrumental way in his breadwinning behavior, in a mutual way in marriage and friendship, and in a vectorial way in parenthood, charitable, and idealistic endeavors. A well-adjusted individual is capable of acting in a reasonably balanced way on all three levels.

Observations of patients brought unexpected yet irresistible conclusions. Some patients acted in an extreme instrumental way, some displayed exaggerated and wholly irrational vectorialism, while the third group swung from one extreme to another in a distortion of mutualism. Hence, three pathological types: the psychopathic hyperinstrumentals, the cyclic-depressive dysmutuals, and the schizoid hypervectorials.

Thus a new theory and classification of mental disorders ensued. This theory, based on observable interactional patterns, is open to empirical test. At the same time, it is isomorphic to a somewhat modified psychoanalytic theory of personality.

A study of families of schizophrenic patients represented an almost uniform pattern. Despite the great variability in life histories, the basic features were always the same. Parent-parent attitude was hostile-instrumental, mother-child attitude was pseudo-vectorial and actually exploitative-instrumental, father-child attitude was seductive or competitive-instrumental. Thus the establishment of a normal child-parent relationship was prevented.

While doing intensive psychotherapy with adults and children in this country, I began to look back into my old notes and papers and case reports from bygone years overseas. I embarked on systematic interviewing with parents of schizophrenics. I sat in on a children's ward in a mental hospital, checking files, observing children, and talking to the personnel. I have supervised several psychotherapists. The results of all this work are given in the present book.

The present book is not a research monograph. Although several research projects are incorporated here, the purpose of this volume is not to report systematic findings but to offer an over-all theory based on thirty years of experience and hundreds of cases, some of them treated, some supervised, some observed. This book organizes the available data obtained by scores of workers and my own observations into one coherent system. It is a hypothetical system and a set of therapeutic proposals.

Certainly this system is full of loopholes and shortcomings, and I shall share my observations and doubts with the reader and point to controversies and inadequacies in available empirical data, including my own.

Yet despite the obvious shortcomings, I feel that this is the right track to be followed. Certainly the data must be more precise, more reliable, and better controlled, and the whole theory exposed to a rigorous empirical test. But, as the proverb says, even the longest road must start from the first step. Thus, let us close the preface and start the book.

BENJAMIN B. WOLMAN

Contents

CHAPTER 1

The Concept of Schizophrenia

1. BASIC IDEAS

Incidence

There has been a widespread reluctance to describe a child as being psychotic. Therefore many euphemistic terms have been used, such as "pseudopsychosis" and "incipient" and "borderline psychosis," to describe children who show a clear pattern of psychotic behavior. However, since the term childhood schizophrenia was introduced, more and more children have been included in this category.

According to Milt (1963), there are approximately 4000 psychotic children in state hospitals, close to 2500 in residential treatment and day care centers, and at least 3000 schizophrenic children are seen in outpatient clinics.

The estimates of childhood schizophrenia run from 100,000 to half a million children. Considering the over-all estimate of the per cent of schizophrenics in the general population, the half-a-million figure does not seem too exaggerated.

Some research workers believe that childhood schizophrenia is not the same clinical entity as schizophrenia in adulthood. However, in longitudinal studies of adult schizophrenics, I have repeatedly discovered the connection between schizophrenia in childhood and adulthood. Of course one must keep in mind that, irrespective of clinical similarities, a schizophrenic child is a child and not an adult.

Schizophrenia does not start in adulthood; it does not resemble Pallas Athena, who sprang as a grown woman in full armor from the head of Zeus. Schizophrenia starts early and grows slowly, warping the emotions and destroying the personality structure from within. In some cases the so-called psychotic breakdown resembles a sudden collapse of a house, and in other cases it is a slow erosion.

1

In either case the downfall is a product of gradual decline and decay.

A retrospective search of the life histories of adult schizophrenics (Wolman, 1957, 1966) reveals various degrees of severity of schizophrenia in childhood. Thus it seems methodologically advisable to attempt to relate the various syndromes of childhood schizophrenia to corresponding syndromes in adult schizophrenia and thereby to establish a research continuum.

Narcissistic Disorders

A concise presentation of Freud's ideas on schizophrenia was given by Fenichel (1945, pages 414-416), who wrote:

> The infant starts out in a state of "primary narcissism" in which the systems of the mental apparatus are not yet differentiated from each other, and in which no objects exist as yet. The differentiation of the ego coincides with the discovery of objects. An ego exists in so far as it is differentiated from objects that are not ego. . . . The schizophrenic has regressed to narcissism; the schizophrenic has lost his objects; the schizophrenic has parted with reality; the schizophrenic's ego has broken down. In schizophrenia the collapse of reality test, the fundamental function of the ego, and the symptoms of "disintegration of the ego" which amount to a severe disruption of the continuity of the personality, likewise can be interpreted as a return to the time when the ego was not yet established or had just begun to be established.

Self-Hypocathexis

Federn (1952), however, assumed a different position regarding schizophrenia. He proposed that all children are born narcissistic, and that it takes both libidinal development through biologically determined stages and learning by environmental experiences to enable the individual to attain some balance between self- and object cathexis. But in instances where parents force the child to renounce narcissism too early and induce the child to take a protective, parental attitude towards them, the normal processes of maturation and learning become disrupted. The child is forced to hypercathect his love objects at the expense of self-cathexis. The end result of this disruption is that the ego becomes so impoverished that it is unable to maintain itself.

Theoretical Considerations

The present volume accepts the Freudian personality model based on (1) the driving instinctual forces of love and hate; (2) the mental strata—the unconscious, preconscious, and conscious; and (3) the mental apparatus—the id, ego, and superego.

The choice of this model has been dictated by several considerations: (1) Freud's personality model enables one to deal with psychological phenomena in psychological terms and also to relate them to somatic phenomena; (2) Freud's developmental stages include both the innate factors of maturation and the environmental forces that facilitate learning, and (3) Freud's theory of personality includes normal and pathological phenomena in one continuum.

Yet the specific approach to the problem of schizophrenia as taken by this book is more related to that of Federn. This position assumes that in well-adjusted individuals there is a *balance of cathexes in oneself and in others* that permits the individual to protect himself and to take care of those he loves. This balance can be disturbed in three major directions. Some individuals develop a narcissistic, morbid self-hypercathexis after they have been seriously thwarted in the development of object cathexis. Others are unable to take care of themselves, due to insufficient self-cathexis and overabundant object cathexis. Still others shift from one extreme to the other (Wolman, 1965b).

Moreover, the terms libido, cathexis, etc., are unobservables; they are theoretical constructs that require empirical, observable, testable counterparts. Such observables, derived from the study of overt interactional processes, are described briefly below.

Classification

The human neonate interacts with parents and other individuals from the day he is born. Unless his organism was impaired by hereditary factors or by prenatal, natal, or postnatal physicochemical noxious factors, the mental disorder is started by his interaction with the social environment.

One may distinguish three patterns of observable social interaction (Wolman, 1956, 1958a, 1960). Whenever an individual enters a social relationship with the objective of having his own needs satisfied, it is an *instrumental social* pattern. The individual is a *taker* and uses others for the satisfaction of his needs. All business relationships are instrumental; a man sells goods, hires service, or looks for a job in order to satisfy his own needs.

The second type of relationship is *mutual,* or mutual acceptance. Whenever an individual enters a social relationship with the objective of *giving and taking,* to satisfy his own needs and to satisfy the needs of others, it is a mutual relationship. Friendship, partnership, and marriage are usually mutual relationships.

Certain relationships belong to the third, *vectorial* type. True charity, i.e., giving without expecting anything in return, is vectorial. So is one's dedication to his religion, homeland, or any other ideal.

The infant-toward-parent relationship is the prototype of instrumentalism; the husband and wife relationship is the prototype of mutualism; the parent-toward-infant relationship is the prototype of vectorialism. The normal adult acts in a balanced manner in all three types of relationships; he is instrumental in his breadwinning activities, mutual in regard to his marital partner, friends, and relatives, and vectorial toward his children and toward those who need his help.

Severe distortion or imbalance in social interaction is indicative of mental disorder. One may, therefore, classify sociogenic mental disorders using overt interactional patterns as a criterion (Wolman, 1965b).

Observing mentally disturbed people, one can discern, despite the diversity of symptoms, three fairly consistent patterns of abnormal social interaction. These patterns are so pervading, so apparent, so easily observable, that they can be used also as diagnostic clues to be applied in Chapter 6.

The Hyperinstrumental Type

Some mentally disturbed individuals are hyperinstrumental. They always want something for nothing; they show no consideration for their fellow men, not even for their own parents, marital partners, or children; they are convinced that the world owes them a living, but that they do not owe anything to anyone in return. They treat life like a bank to be robbed or an oil field to be exploited, and have no love for anyone except themselves. They feel sorry for themselves only, and believe in their own impeccable innocence.

The *hyperinstrumental type* corresponds to what is usually called the psychopath or sociopath. The libido of the psychopath is self-hypercathected, for he has never outgrown the primary narcissism. His object relations are exploitative, primitive-instrumental, mostly on the oral-cannibalistic level. In hyperinstrumentals, the destrudo is always object-directed. The hyperinstrumental type views others as enemies bound to devour him, unless he devours them. He treats weak people the way the wolf treats sheep, but he acts in a cowardly way toward the strong ones.

The hyperinstrumental type has practically no superego, has no moral principles and no human obligations. He does not trust people, thus he often develops paranoid delusions. Since his libido is excessively self-cathected, he overdoes in caring for himself and the mildest ache causes hypochondriac fears.

Dysmutual Type

The second type is an epitomy of inconsistency. Sometimes the dysmutuals overdo in love, and sometimes they feel no love for others and are as selfish as the hyperinstrumentals. When the dysmutuals love, they expect their love objects to return love with a high interest rate; when in love they are hyperaffectionate, showering protectiveness and tenderness, and are ready for any self-sacrifice. However, when not repaid in full, their assumed great and unselfish love turns into a selfish, brutal hostility. But not only does their object love turn easily into hostility; the same also happens with their attitude toward themselves. Usually they love themselves very much, but often their self-directed love turns into hate and leads to suicidal attempts. Their changing, cyclic moods reflect their libido and destrudo imbalance. When they feel loved, they believe themselves to be great, strong, wonderful, and their mood is elated. When they feel rejected, they believe themselves to be weak, small, destitute, and hostile, and their mood is depressed. These fluctuations of mood gave rise to the name *manic depressives*. The dysmutual type is torn by exaggerated feelings of love and hate toward others and themselves. In a loving mood they are Dr. Jekyll; in a hating mood they are Mr. Hyde. Since none of these moods is lasting, they give the impression of being insincere. Actually, they swing from extreme honesty to dishonesty, from love to hate, from heroism to cowardice.

Hypervectorial Type

The hypervectorial disturbed individuals are extreme opposites to the first type. They are hypervectorial even in situations in which people are usually instrumental. They are always ready to give, to protect, and to sacrifice themselves. In their childhood they did not act as all other children did, i.e., in a naturally instrumental way, but as if they were the *protectors of their parents.* As adults they seem to believe that they owe everything to the world and no one owes them anything. Unless they are badly deteriorated, they seem to believe that life is an obligation to be honored, a ritual to be followed, or a mission to be fulfilled. They have sympathy for everyone except for themselves. When they love someone, they are exceedingly loyal, but also overprotective, domineering, and despotic in their overprotectiveness. When their exaggerated self-controls fail, they may regress into autistic seclusion.

The name hypervectorialism covers all that is called schizophrenia and related conditions. The formation of symptoms in hypervectorialism mainly offers primary gain. The hypervectorials believe that they are not as good as they should be and fear their own hostility. Their libido is object hypercathected and their destrudo overrepressed. Their superego is overgrown and dictatorial, hence their behavior is often self-righteous.

A description of personality dynamics in adult schizophrenia follows.

2. SCHIZOPHRENIA IN ADULTS

Personality Dynamics in Schizophrenia

The preschizophrenic starts his life as any other neonate in a state of primary narcissism with all his libido invested in himself and all his destrudo (aggressive energy) ready to be directed against threatening objects. In a normal development, the loving and protecting (vectorial) parental attitude enables the child to grow and develop normal instrumental, mutual, and vectorial attitudes. The preschizophrenic child, however, realizes that his parents are not protective and that, therefore, unless he protects them he may lose them. The schizophrenic paradox reads as follows: "I want to live, but I must sacrifice my own life to protect those upon whom my survival depends." This attitude leads to an abundant, hypervectorial cathexis of the child's libido in his parents and extreme efforts on his part to inhibit his self-protective outbursts of destrudo directed against those whom he must protect at his own expense. The schizophrenic fears that his inadequate love of parents and loss of control over his own hostility may kill them and then he will be lost forever.

Thus, schizophrenia is essentially an *irrational struggle for survival*. The fear of losing the love object forces the individual to care more for the object than he does for himself. This hypervectorial object cathexis reduces the individual's own resources and prevents adequate self-cathexis (cf. Federn, 1952). When the shrinking amount of libido left for self-cathexis is unable to protect the individual, the destrudo takes over.

As has been previously mentioned, the toilet training stage is the one during which the normal child develops a sense of mutuality. Feces are the first indisputable possession of the child, and toilet training introduces the first gift-giving relationship and the first sacrifice. The child learns to postpone immediate satisfaction for a future gratification derived from delayed elimination and maternal approval.

The preschizophrenic, however, never receives whole-hearted approval, for no matter what he gives it is not enough. His efforts do not satisfy his mother, and his true or alleged imperfections are held responsible for the mother's true or imaginary ailments. Thus, he continually feels that he must strive harder in his efforts to love and protect her.

The preschizophrenic learns early to sacrifice his *pleasure principle* without obtaining an adequate *reality principle*. Normally, the infant learns to postpone immediate gratification and pleasure for a future, a better, and a less threatening one. This is the reality principle. But the *preschizophrenic is forced to renounce his pleasure principle without any further compensation*. He is forced to sacrifice his own needs for those of others, and pushed into a hypervectorial position.

This self-hypocathexis is often disastrous for the individual, and one of the impending signs of this disaster is the breaking through of destrudo. It is here assumed that libido and destrudo are two types of the same mental energy and are mutually transferable. Libido is the higher, destrudo the lower energy, and when libido fails in serving survival destrudo takes over.

In brief, there are three main causes precipitating outbursts of hostility. When the individual supply of *libido is exhausted* he becomes hostile in an effort to protect himself. Hostility is also provoked when the individual's *hypervectorial libidinal cathexis are turned down* by his love object. Finally, in an effort to protect himself from the devastating effect of his self-directed hostility in the form of guilt and self-recrimination, the individual may *project* his hostility against others. Yet outbursts of hostility represent a threat to the individual's parental pseudo protectors, and thus the fear of his own destructive power forms an important theme of the schizophrenic's preoccupations and, in some cases, hallucinations.

The Unconscious and the Conscious

According to Freud, the entire id belongs to the province or layer of unconscious, while only parts of the ego and superego are unconscious. Normally, unconscious wishes are partly repressed, partly sublimated, and partly incorporated in, and subordinated to, the conscious purposes of the ego.

The flow of unconscious impulses becomes dangerous to the total personality structure only when the conscious ego lacks the power to harness them or put a check on them in the ways mentioned above. And this is precisely what happens in schizophrenia.

The schizophrenic process is characterized by efforts to overcontrol unconscious impulses. A failure of these efforts leads to a full-blown psychotic breakdown. The desperate repressive efforts taken by the preschizophrenic to control his unconscious are made necessary by two major factors.

First, weakness of the ego is common to all preschizophrenics. The ego grows and thrives on contacts with reality, on testing reality, and on playing an active part in interindividual relationships, through contacts which are limited in the life of the preschizophrenic.

The second reason for the increased fear of the unconscious is the content and intensity of the unconscious wishes. The peculiar family situation strengthens and magnifies the unconscious incestuous impulses. These impulses, latent in all individuals, have been stirred up, fomented, and brought to a pitch by the unfortunate interindividual relationships in schizogenic families.

Even more threatening than incestuous impulses, however, are the aggressive impulses. Parental attitudes usually create some degree of resentment in children; part of this resentment is repressed, part acted out in little rebellious acts against the parents, part sublimated, and part stored in the superego. There is much more of this resentment in the forced hypervectorial development than in a normal childhood. Furthermore, the preschizophrenic is much too involved emotionally to be able to sublimate and too afraid of losing his parents to act out his hostility. As a result, he carries the dynamite of destrudo, partly repressed and partly stored in the superego.

This hypocathected impoverished ego has to mobilize all its resources to prevent explosions of pent-up hostility. The typical schizophrenic either regresses gradually in a slow deterioration process through the neurotic, character neurotic, latent psychotic, manifest psychotic, and dementive stages, or skips some stages in a sudden psychotic breakdown.

The story of schizophrenia is the story of the ego's desperate struggle to control the unconscious impulses. The results of that struggle will determine whether a stop will be made on a milder level or whether the individual will go all the way down toward a complete dismemberment of personality.

Id, Ego, and Superego

The superego develops out of fear of parental punishment and need for protection and affection. The child "internalizes" parental prohibitions and, through introjection, identifies with the parental figures. Parental actions and attitudes, as perceived by the child, become an important factor in shaping his personality. Conformity with parental demands lays the foundations for the social adjustment of the individual and for his acceptance of the cultural value system of his environment.

In the schizophrenic personality structure, the superego plays a peculiar role. The superego usually represents "the voice of parents" and their moral standards as perceived by the child. The superego may be irrational, childish, rigid, unrealistic, and inconsiderate of real circumstances. The mental energy of the superego includes both libido and destrudo; the child "introjects" the love object that causes him so much frustration. The amount of destrudo invested in the introjected parental images corresponds to the degree of resentment the child has had toward the parents.

The superego of the latent schizophrenic is not intentionally destructive, but its influence can have a damaging effect on the ego, and its demands for absolute obedience and submission from the ego impose a totalitarian slavery on the ego, forcing it to reduce its contact with the outer world and secure a strict control over the instinctual demands of the id (Wolman, 1957; 1966).

Normally the ego accepts most of the moral guidance of the superego, exercises a moderate and rational control over the id, and keeps an eye on the outer world, the reality. In a schizophrenic type of development, the superego very early assumes absolute control over the ego and insists on a severe repression of the demands of the id.

The ego may be forced to neglect its contacts with the outer world when all its resources become involved in the fight against the id and conflicts with the superego. This deficient contact with the outer world deprives the ego of its most important source of guidance and encouragement. The preschizophrenic child is so preoccupied with his mother that he is forced to reduce his object cathexes of school, studies, other children, and entertainment.

There is no reward for loyalty to the superego. The ego fights desperately against the id impulses and erects rigid barriers in the form of rituals and compulsions, in submission to the severely criticizing, humiliating, punishing, and rigid superego rules. The morale of the ego, the self-esteem, becomes badly impaired, and the ego fights with less and less courage; this, in turn, invites more and more criticism from the despotic superego.

The Dependence-Independence Syndrome

Decision making is always a great problem for schizophrenics because no matter what they decide, their superego will criticize the decision. The conflict usually begins in childhood. Normally a child learns to overcome the id impulses by ego controls assisted by parental prohibitions that become internalized and form the superego. In most cases, these prohibitions correspond to common sense and, resultingly, strengthen the ego.

Parental prohibitions and admonitions in schizogenic families (cf. Lidz et al., 1957, 1958, 1960) are often at odds with logic and common sense and offer no help in adjustment to real life. Moreover, schizogenic mothers are constantly tearing their children down, making them feel inadequate.

No wonder preschizophrenics are overdependent and unable to make their own decisions. They are, however, often rebellious, torn between the superego's dictated overdependence and the normal, ego-inspired struggle for independence. Hence, the dependence-independence oscillation; while wishing to get direct guidance, preschizophrenics resent being pushed and forced (cf. Whitehorn, 1952). Yet at times they arrive at a particular conclusion, and may stubbornly stick to it. When their superego approves of the ego, as when occasionally mother supported the child's decision, this makes the preschizophrenic feel sure of himself and self-righteous.

The Dictatorial Superego

In some cases the tyranny of the superego is so severe that the ego tries to preserve some self-identity by distorting reality or giving it up altogether. The ego regresses to archaic modes of perception which are slanted to fit the demands of the superego, just as the child had to accept the irrational parental ideas. Among these modes are projections, ideas of references, and delusions and hallucinations.

Projections are irrational defenses of the ego against the attacks of the superego. Ideas of references point to an effort of the ego to externalize the pressures of the superego. When the despotic superego presses the ego very hard, the failing ego may perceive the superego's manipulations as if they were coming from without.

Schizophrenics have delusions and hallucinations of power, never weakness. Overidentification with parents gives the superego the feeling of enormous power. Patients with an overgrown superego perceive themselves as a superparent, God-Father, creator-protector, or judge-destroyer of the world.

The weaker the ego, the more aggressive is the superego. The more the superego attacks, the weaker the ego becomes. The superego criticizes the ego for its failure to assume an absolute and perfect control over the id, but attacks from the superego on the ego render any control of the id impossible.

The failing ego loses its grip on reality and its control over the id. The vehement impulses, sexual and aggressive, break through, leaving the ego each time more defenseless than before. The ego, attacked by both the id and the superego, may disintegrate and give up contact with reality.

Role of the Ego

The severity of schizophrenia depends mostly on the degree of the damage caused to the ego by the premature hypervectorial object cathexis. Taking this point of view, it seems evident that, all other factors being equal, the earlier schizophrenia starts, the more serious it is. Early childhood schizophrenia, or *vectoriasis praecocissima,* is thus the most severe disorder in the group of schizophrenias. It is a failure of the ego that has not yet developed. Of course the time factor is not the only factor, for even the well-developed ego can disintegrate when it is exposed to exceedingly severe blows.

To summarize, the ego in a schizophrenic-type disorder suffers two initial setbacks: deficient self-cathexis caused by an inadequate supply of energy, resulting from a lavish object hypercathexis, and an overwhelming job of protecting life while exposed to unbearable pressure from the environment (parents) and from within (the superego and id).

Emergency Situations

It has been observed that schizophrenics often improve in the face of a real emergency, when in serious external danger, or when undergoing a severe physical illness. The interpretation of these well-known phenomena depends on the theory of balance of cathexes. A serious threat to life forces a withdrawal of object cathexis and restoration of a normal libido balance. This fact can perhaps shed light on the positive reactions to shock treatment; it is possible that the organism responds to a severe shock with a reversal of cathexes. However, not all such individuals are capable of reinvesting their libido in themselves, and at a certain level of deterioration even a lethal danger cannot help.

Reality Testing

Schizophrenia can strike people at any level of intellectual development and any I.Q., and there is no evidence of relationship between schizophrenia and mental development.

It has also been said that, no matter what their intelligence, the intellectual functioning of schizophrenics shows certain peculiarities. As a result of an unusual mobilization of the ego, preschizophrenics frequently display a great deal of precision in their thinking. Many of them are diligent students and most conscientious workers. However, their concentrated effort is frequently hampered by emotional factors and their performance is rather uneven. When they deteriorate, the oscillations in performance become spectacular, with several areas being blocked out, while in one or two fields the individual performs unusually well, as if whatever was left of the overmobilized ego became cathected there.

Latent schizophrenics display an unusual perceptiveness, intuition, and empathy. The preschizophrenic child is so fearful for his parents that he spends a tremendous amount of energy watching them closely and trying to gain clues to their emotional state. Moreover, since the preschizophrenic expects the worst, his oversensitized perception is often colored by his own worries and fears, and quite often confused with paranoid projections.

Emotionality

Schizophrenics have been characterized as highly emotional and dramatic and also as lacking affect, shallow and withdrawn, and both descriptions can be observed.

Schizophrenia is a disbalance in the basic emotions of love and hate. When too much love has been stirred up, brought to a boiling point, and given away in vain, a violent hate can be elicited. Schizophrenics love and hate intensely and fear their own vehement emotions. An extraordinary effort to control emotions and their volcano-like eruptions are symptomatic for schizophrenia.

The preschizophrenic child, as any other child, is prone to express his emotions without delay. Outbursts of both joyful love and temper tantrums, feelings of bliss and utter despair, are normal behavior patterns of infants. Gradually they learn to control their emotions.

The preschizophrenic child is almost incessantly overstimulated emotionally. His parents do not exercise control, and thus he is unable to learn from them. Moreover, he is met with anger and retaliation whenever he does express himself. The threat of punishment forces him to become rigid in his emotional control and fear his own feelings.

Schizophrenics may therefore appear cold and detached, while inwardly they are on the verge of an eruption. Most latent schizophrenics shun close human relations. They fear becoming emotionally involved and withdraw from intense social contacts. They do not allow themselves to respond to human warmth for fear of repetition of the relationship with their parents. Thus they appear to others as aloof, cold, shallow, uninterested in other people, and self-centered. They rigidly control their emotions to the extent that these emotions become repressed, isolated, and displaced.

Yet at times these emotions break through. Preschizophrenics, as a rule, are tactful, thoughtful, and considerate. They would rather attack themselves than others. However, as soon as the ego loses its grip over the impulses, pent-up hostility comes violently to the fore. Handling of hostility and of defenses against hostility, therefore, becomes a major therapeutic task.

Control of Motility

Abnormalities in schizophrenic motor behavior are apparently caused by the efforts of the ego to overcontrol the system, and the eventual failure of these efforts. Preschizophrenics often appear to be well-functioning, poised, precise in their movements, harmonious, and calm, while inwardly they are tense and aggitated. When faced with a problem or task, they may exercise perfect muscular and general self-control, frequently followed by such aftereffects as crying spells and excessive fatigue.

These swings from overcontrol to loss of control are typical of the schizophrenic process. In normal circumstances the ego plays a significant role in motor coordination. On the preschizophrenic level overcoordination approximates perfection, but as the individual deteriorates several motor symptoms appear, among them all kinds of weird postures, tics, rigidity, clonic and tonic stupors, echolalias, echopraxias, and other disturbances of speech and mannerisms. These well-known symptoms of schizophrenia point up the inner conflicts in the control of the motor apparatus which probably begins with fears generated by toilet training. The mother demands that the child achieve absolute control, and he is terrified that he will not meet her demands.

Motor disturbances also evidence the cryptic language of the unconscious. Some schizophrenic mannerisms, such as sucking, rocking, etc., are signs of infantile regression. Others, such as echopraxia and echolalia, probably express identification with the environment. Still others, such as self-mutilation, are expressions of self-directed hostility that can no longer be controlled by the failing ego.

Loss of Self-Esteem

Self-esteem is a product of the relationship between the superego and the ego. When the superego tears the ego down, the individual experiences feelings of inferiority and inadequacy. When the superego approves of the ego, a feeling of power and elation ensues.

It must be remembered that the feeling of power has tremendous psychological importance. Feeling strong enables one to become generous while feeling weak forces one into a hostile attitude toward the threatening world.

Sullivan displayed keen insight when he wrote that schizophrenia is a catastrophe in self-esteem (1947, 1962). The tormenting feelings of one's own worthlessness, guilt, and inadequacy are common to all schizophrenia. On a prepsychotic level, schizophrenics doubt their appearance, intelligence, and honesty and blame themselves for whatever hardships they have had. When seriously deteriorated, they do not care about their physical appearance, their jobs, income, food, or health. Moreover, they often provoke fights, expecting defeat and accepting it as a deserved punishment.

The Id

The id, said Freud, is a "cauldron of seething excitement," the prime source of all mental energies. The id does not change. It is always the same source of unbounded, fluid energy, seeking quick discharge in accordance with the pleasure principle.

Furthermore, the id is blind. Most animals have an instinctual faculty for sensing oncoming danger. In human beings the id does not offer such protection; the ego is the protector of the organism. It seems that the id does sense danger, but it does not react in a manner best suited to protect the organism in the complex situations of human civilization. A scared infant screams, fights, and turns red or pale. A scared adult seeks protection by an ego-controlled and rationally executed fight or flight.

The feelings of an oncoming danger are not identical with a logical prediction of danger; the former is a function of the id. Although schizophrenics may react to danger in a highly irrational and futile way, there is no doubt that they frequently sense the oncoming danger and become much upset by it. Hence, they may pose a sort of "premonition," similar to the tense behavior displayed by some animals on the eve of a flood, earthquake, or other catastrophe.

Many symptoms of schizophrenia reflect the rule of the unconscious superego with its tyrannical, self-righteous methods. Most hallucinations are superego hallucinations, reflecting the wish of the schizophrenic to be omnipotent superparents. In severe hebephrenic and dementive cases the id takes over. There are no more guilt feelings, no more considerations, no more fear of consequences. Both the ego and the superego are shattered, and the id is in complete control.

Somatic Factors

Many researchers have attempted to prove that schizophrenia is caused by somatic factors, but the present theory proposes that the somatic changes found in schizophrenia are of a psychosomatic nature. Furthermore, these psychosomatic changes can be caused either by conditioning or by cathexis or both (Wolman, 1966).

Most psychoanalysts relate somatic symptoms to hypochondriasis and self-hypercathexis (Alexander and Flagg, 1965). The present interpretation of these phenomena goes in the opposite direction and points to an *inadequate self-cathexis*. The hypothesis of somatic symptoms of hypocathected bodily organs completes the theory of *schizophrenia* as a *sociopsychosomatic disorder*. Noxious *environmental* (social) *factors* cause disbalance in interindividual cathexes of libido and destrudo, which in turn introduce serious changes in the total personality structure (psychological factors). The personality disorders cause, in turn, somatic changes, either by psychosomatic transformations of deficiency in mental energy into organic deficiencies, or by the process of conditioning (Wolman, 1967).

Russian studies in conditioning (Bykov, 1957) point to such a possibility, in that they have shown that higher order conditioning is applicable to inner organs. Psychologically induced changes in heart beat, rate of metabolism, and circulation of blood are not limited to Charcot's hysterics. They are common to all humans, inclusive of schizophrenics, and can be induced by conditioning.

Schizophrenia is here defined as an effort to survive on an evolutionary lower level of living. If this definition is accepted, it is clear that the psychosomatic changes are a continuation of this downward adjustment process. At this point, one cannot but vaguely speculate in regard to neurological and biochemical counterparts of this process, but all the observed phenomena point to a general process of *lowering of the level of living of schizophrenics in order to preserve life itself.* (See Chapter 2.)

Symptomatology

The approach taken in this book is based on a division of schizophrenic symptoms according to ego strength. The *ego protective* symptoms indicate the struggle of the ego to retain control over the unconscious impulses. Defense mechanisms, such as repression, rationalization, reaction formation, etc., and varieties of neurotic symptoms, such as compulsions, phobias, etc., belong to this category. Furthermore, then *ego protective* symptoms may postpone or even prevent psychotic breakdown.

When these symptoms fail, however, a series of *ego deficiency* symptoms start, indicating an insidious or sudden collapse of the ego. Loss of contact with reality, paranoid delusions, hallucinations, ideas of reference, inability to control unconscious impulses, violence, stupor, depersonalization, as well as motor and speech disturbances belong to the category of ego deficiency symptoms.

In describing preschizophrenic and schizophrenic syndromes, it seems most feasible to use the continuum approach starting from almost normal behavior and going toward the most severe forms. On this continuum one may distinguish five levels of mental disorders, namely, neurosis, character neurosis, latent psychosis, manifest psychosis, and dementive level.

In hypervectorial (overabundant cathexes of others and thus self-neglect), that is, schizo-type, disorders, the neurotic stage includes phobic, neurasthenic, and obsessive-compulsive patterns. The schizoid character neurosis corresponds to what is usually called the schizoid personality. The next level in schizophrenic deterioration is latent schizophrenia, which represents the individual who is still in control but who is on the verge of breakdown. Next comes manifest schizophrenia, called *vectoriasis praecox* (Wolman, 1957; 1966). The last, dementive level represents the end of decline and a complete collapse of personality structure. All five levels represent an ever-growing disbalance of cathexis of sexual and hostile impulses.

The decline of the controlling force of the ego is the most significant determinant of each level. As long as the ego exercises control, it is neurosis. When the ego comes to terms with the symptoms, it is character neurosis. When the ego is on the verge of collapse, it is latent psychosis. When the ego fails, it is manifest psychosis, or full-blown schizophrenia in one of its four syndromes. Finally, a complete dilapidation of the ego and behavior on the id level is typical of the severely deteriorated, dementive stage.

The four syndromes of manifest schizophrenia can also be presented on a continuum of increasing severity starting from paranoid schizophrenia, though catatonic, hebephrenic, and simple deterioration syndromes. In paranoid schizophrenia the defeated ego protects itself against superego assaults by projection and assumes that its own hostility is merely a defense against assaults from without. In catatonic schizophrenia the superego takes over, paralyzing practically all activities; occasionally, when the id breaks through, catatonic fury replaces catatonic stupor. In the hebephrenic syndrome the triumphant id rules, breaking all inhibitions of the ego and superego. The simple deterioration syndrome is, however, the most severe one, for in these cases desire to live is gone. Moreover, if schizophrenia is a "regression for survival" and a withdrawal from normal life, the simple deterioration cases represent, as it were, the "pure" schizophrenia. Most schizophrenics, when locked up for years in a mental institution, deteriorate severely and end up in a dementive state (Arieti, 1955; Wolman, 1966).

Paranoid Syndrome

Not every manifest schizophrenic represents a clear-cut clinical picture, but most of them display one pattern more than another. Several cases start with paranoid symptoms and end up as catatonics. Paranoid tendencies, as a rule, are present in all schizophrenics, for all schizophrenics use this mechanism to ward off the panic feeling stemming from their own hostility.

In the paranoid manifest schizophrenia, projection serves the purpose of alleviating the superego's pressure and the resulting guilt feeling. This maneuver is unconscious, and it badly damages reality testing; it is wholly irrational and, thus, psychotic. Projection mechanisms can be partly used on neurotic levels; on manifest psychotic levels they play, however, an outstanding role.

Paranoid ideas of reference relate to the fear that this maneuver may be discovered. It usually starts in childhood when the pre-schizophrenic comes to think that his mother always knows about his intended transgressions. What actually happens gives him the impression that mother is always right. Since mother is always critical, he has to come to the conclusion that he is bad and mother was reading his thoughts. She knows that he has "bad thoughts."

Catatonic Syndrome

In paranoid schizophrenia a morbid compromise is established between the ego and superego. The failing ego has lost control over the id, but it has somehow mollified superego's criticism by giving up reality testing and ascribing sexual and aggressive impulses to the environment. In catatonic schizophrenia the superego takes over the control of the motor apparatus also. Rigid passivity and complete submissiveness are imposed on the organism. The individual renounces his own desires and is all subservience and obedience.

When a catatonic imitates the posture and the movements of whoever addresses him or when he mechanically accepts a certain posture, it is an expression of an infantile, automatic obedience. He does what in his regressed mind he believes he is supposed to do. Catatonic mannerisms and actions like echolalia and echopraxia are signs of submission. A catatonic was told in childhood he was supposed to do what mother did; this was the only way he could be a "good child" and please mother. Mother used to tell him that he was no good; life seemingly confirmed her opinion. Everyone was against him: school, teachers, mates, neighbors, friends, strangers. Everything wrong had to happen to him because he was bad. Being bad might lead to loss of mother and his own death. The schizophrenia paradox, "in order to live he has to give up his own independent life," leads to catatonic passivity and to a renunciation of his own desires and identity.

Hebephrenic Syndrome

In hebephrenia "the ego undertakes no activity for the purpose of defending itself but, beset by conflicts, 'lets itself go.' If the present is unpleasant, the ego withdraws to the past; if the newer types of adaptation fail, it takes refuge in older ones, in the infantile ones of passive receptivity and even, perhaps, in intrauterine ones. If a more differentiated type of living becomes too difficult, it is given up in favor of a more or less vegetative existence. Campbell called it 'schizophrenic surrender.' " (Fenichel, 1945, p. 423.)

The hebephrenic behavioral peculiarities stem from the confusion of developmental strata, learned patterns, and early schizophrenic elements. Hebephrenics can be as suspicious as paranoids and as vehement as catatonics; they lack, however, the ego protective symptoms of partial reality testing of the paranoid schizophrenics and the stuporous defenses of the catatonics. They are easily provoked into uncontrollable outbursts of rage directed against self and others. The provocation is usually a true, or believed to be true, unfriendly gesture coming from the environment.

The disturbances in reality testing, cognitive functions, reasoning, and thought processes are most pronounced. Hebephrenics experience delusions of grandeur, hallucinate frequently, have ideas of reference, and paranoid fears. They regress to primary prelogical and irrational ways of thinking. Their reasoning lacks purpose and consistency, is full of condensations and distortions, and their associations follow verbal, phonetic, or any other irrelevant clue. Their giggling, laughing, anger, or apprehension bear witness to their lack of contact with reality and reflect primary processes.

Simple Deterioration Syndrome

The "simple deterioration" type has often been called "simple" and, as such, believed to be mild. This is, however, not the case, and the simple deterioration means that the organism has given up its fight for survival and the main objective of the ego, self-protection, has been lost. The onset is usually insidious, gradual, and slow. The origins may go far back into early childhood. Most of the simple deterioration cases have a long history of maladjustment, social withdrawal, and daydreaming; in their earliest years they displayed some autistic features, shyness, inability to do things on their own, lack of interest, lack of initiative, depressive moods, and a peculiar type of docile, passive, overdependent behavior, with occasional crying spells and irritability periods.

This renunciation of one's own narcissistic pleasures and sacrificing of everything for the parents is perhaps the purest form of *vectoriasis praecox.* In all other forms of schizophrenia there is an inner fight between the normal self-preservation drive and the desire to protect the protectors. In the simple deterioration form there is very little, if any, fight. The ego gives up its main task. The individual gives away everything, and there is nothing left to keep him alive: no interest, no ambition, no desire to live. The profound decline of sensitivity to pain makes one less capable of survival, less ready to avoid injury.

Dementive Stage

In terms of personality dynamics, dementia represents decay and destruction of a human personality structure. Apparently in the fifth or dementive level of schizophrenia, there is just id. Ego and superego do not interfere, perhaps are nonexistent. Imagine a neonate, and imagine that he grows physically and lives on pleasure principle (i.e., the principle of immediate gratification of needs). Repetitive movements, aimless activity, mannerisms, no control of bowels and bladder remind one of severe mental defectives.

Childhood Schizophrenia: A Reversal of Adult Schizophrenia

A schizophrenic child is a child, and growth and maturational processes complicate the clinical picture. As a result, there are several schizo-type behavioral patterns in childhood, depending on the age of the child, sex, severity of damage, level of development, specific family influences, etc.

One important distinction should be made when attempting to relate childhood schizophrenia to adult schizophrenia. Schizophrenia in adulthood is a failure of the impoverished ego. The ego has lost most of its resources in object cathexis, has been hard pressed ("overdemanded") by the superego to control its id, failed in that, and finally is unable to control the id and ceases to be the steering wheel of the organism. In childhood schizophrenic disorders, the ego has never had the chance to assume that role. Schizophrenia in infancy or *vectoriasis praecocissima is a mental catastrophy that takes place even before the ego has the opportunity to grow and to assert control over the id.* It is not easy, therefore, to divide this earliest point of schizophrenia into the clinical syndromes, such as catatonic, paranoid, etc.

The symptomatology of schizophrenia in adults has been presented in order of increasing severity ending in the dementive level (Wolman, 1966). Analysis of the symptomatology of infantile schizophrenia is made in reverse order, starting with the most severe syndromes. The logic of such an order is obvious. In regard to adults, the assumption is that personality structure is regressed; in childhood schizophrenia, the growth has been prevented.

As a rule, the earlier the damage is caused, the more it affects the personality. Accordingly, the following types or degrees of severity of childhood schizophrenia are closely related to the age of onset of the damage.

The first and most severe level, *pseudo-amentive schizophrenia,* roughly corresponds to dementive schizophrenia in adults, the last and most severe level of regression. The second and slightly less severe level is *autistic schizophrenia,* which corresponds to simple deterioration and hebephrenia in adults. The third level, in order of decreasing severity, is *symbiotic schizophrenia,* more or less corresponding to catatonia. The fourth level, *aretic schizophrenia,* corresponds to some extent to the adult paranoid schizophrenic.

The proposed five types of infantile schizophrenia correspond to five stages and manners in which the hypervectorial disorder was produced. Pseudo-amentive childhood schizophrenia is formed on a preverbal, preego formation level. The four other types are formed slightly later, but all of them originate in the first two years of life.

Childhood schizophrenia follows the general schizophrenic principle of downward adjustment or regression for survival. All stages and phases of the hypervectorial disorders follow the same main principles of giving up of one's libidinal resources and, as a result, impoverishment of one's ego.

Schizophrenia in childhood is even more variated than in adult years. When a storm breaks young trees and saplings, no one can predict how each tree will look afterward. Some may be cut in two; some, fortunately, may lose only a few branches; some may survive the damage, while others may be completely destroyed, uprooted, or blown away.

All schizophrenic children are children whose childhood has been taken away—they are *children without childhood,* their *vectoriasis* (schizophrenia) is *praecosissima.*

CHAPTER 2

Etiologic Determinants

1. HISTORICAL REMARKS

As early as in 1812, Benjamin Rush described childhood psychosis in his textbook of psychiatry, the first psychiatric textbook published in the United States. Two of the children described by Rush bit their mothers. Rush interpreted this "madness" as a result of some instability and frequent excitation in the cortex.

In the nineteenth century several psychiatrists and neurologists mentioned mental disorders in childhood and described epilepsy, mental deficiency, delinquency, and various types of insanity. In 1906, five years before publication of E. Bleuler's classic *Dementia Praecox of the Group of Schizophrenias,* Sante de Sanctis described childhood schizophrenia, calling it *dementia praecocissima.* De Sanctis believed that *dementia praecocissima* was a psychosis connected with puberty, and his ideas have been widely accepted. The occurrence of schizophrenia before puberty was considered extremely rare. However, it should be remembered that both Bleuler and Kraepelin stated that at least 25 per cent of schizophrenic cases have started in childhood years.

Observation of the symptoms of childhood schizophrenia has received much more attention than research in etiology. Research and treatment techniques for childhood disorders had not been developed, preventing any real isolation of the complex, often inconsistent, and seemingly contradictory symptoms of childhood schizophrenia. Lack of an adequately elaborated developmental approach to childhood disorders handicapped researchers and practitioners who dealt with the children.

The gradually growing awareness of the magnitude of the problem and progress in research in psychopathology has led to the development of a variety of techniques and theories. Potter in 1933 defined childhood schizophrenia and initiated the controversy of

23

whether it is progressive from childhood to adulthood or reactive to a certain environment or situation. Kanner described early infantile autism as a reaction to cold and unresponsive parents (refrigerator parents). Withdrawal from reality, caused by a peculiar mother-infant relationship, was stressed by several authors. Paul Schilder and Melanie Klein interpreted the etiology of childhood schizophrenia in light of psychoanalytic theory. Melanie Klein attributed childhood schizophrenia to the child's inability to project the introjected "bad" objects.

Schilder further combined the psychoanalytic and neurological points of view and contributed to the understanding of interaction of embryological and psychological factors. He developed the concept of "body image" with respect to the individual's ability to function socially and physically in the world. The concept of normal personality development and the pathological deviations in schizophrenia have been elaborated by Lauretta Bender. Bender related schizophrenia to "maturational lag."

At the present time scores of research workers are studying the various aspects of the highly complex childhood schizophrenia.

2. GENETICS

Kallmann's Data

All mental disorders are either inherited or acquired. The inherited disorders are produced by pathological genes; thus they should be called *genosomatogenic*. Disorders acquired through interaction between the organism and its physical surroundings, and caused by noxious physicochemical agents are *ecosomatogenic*. Mental disorders caused by interaction with a noxious social environment are *sociogenic* or *sociopsychogenic*.

Research in etiology of childhood schizophrenia must examine all possible factors.

Many research workers believe that schizophrenia is an inherited disorder. The leading proponent of the inheritance theory of schizophrenia is F. J. Kallmann (1946, 1953, 1962) who found that children with one schizophrenic parent have 16.4 per cent probability of becoming schizophrenic, while children with two schizophrenic parents have 69.1 per cent probability. Kallmann's comparison of fraternal and identical twins showed that, where one fraternal twin has developed schizophrenia, there was a 16.4 per cent probability that the other twin will also become schizophrenic, while identical twins have an 86.2 per cent chance of both becoming schizophrenic. In a study of 691 twins, Kallmann found in dizygotic twins concordance with schizophrenia in 14.7 per cent of the cases, as compared to 77.6 to 81.5 per cent in monozygotic twins. This higher percentage of 81.5 per cent refers to twins who have been together for five years prior to their breakdown. Therefore Kallmann concluded that "inheritance of schizophrenia follows a biological genetic pattern." (1946, p. 318.) Kallmann, however, did not exclude the role of environmental factors. He wrote (1953) that schizophrenia is "the result of intricate interaction of varying genetic and environmental factors."

Kallmann believes that schizophrenia is caused by a single recessive genetic mechanism with 70 per cent penetrance. In Kallmann's studies the concordance rates for nonseparated and separated monozygotic twins are 91.5 and 77.6 per cent respectively. The difference of 13.9 per cent militates for partial environmental influences. According to Kallmann, the data for concordance rates for dizygotic twins and siblings are 14.5 and 14.2 per cent respectively.

In a study entitled "Genetic Studies of Preadolescent Schizophrenia," Kallmann and Roth (1956) explored six pairs of dizygotic twins and 12 pairs of monozygotic twins below 15 years of age, and two pairs of dizygotic and three monozygotic at age 15 and over. The uncorrected rates for the dizygotic were 17.1 per cent and for the monozygotic 70.6 per cent. However, the ratio of schizophrenic and schizoid children in good homes was 4 per cent, in fair homes 14 per cent, in poor homes 30 per cent, and in broken homes 52 per cent.

The following is a tabular summary of Kallmann's studies of expectancy of schizophrenia (Kallmann, 1962):

One-egg twins	86.2%
Two-egg twins	14.5%
Siblings	14.2%
Half-siblings	7.1%
General population	0.85%

TABLE 1

Variations in the Schizophrenia Rates of Siblings and Twin Partners According to Sex and the Similarity or Dissimilarity in Environment

	Siblings of Twin Index Cases			Dizygotic Co-Twins			Monozygotic Co-Twins		
	Male	Female	Total Number	Male	Female	Total Number	Separated	Non-separated	Total Number
Same sex	1.59	16.3	16.1	17.4	17.7	17.6	77.6	91.5	85.8
Opposite sex	12.5	12.0	12.3	10.5	10.2	10.3	—	—	—
Total number	14.0	14.5	14.3	14.3	14.9	14.7	77.6	91.5	85.8

Adapted from Kallmann, F. J. The genetic theory of schizophrenia. *Amer. J. Psychiat.*, 1946, *103*, p. 316.

Altshuler (1957) confirmed Kallmann's findings, stressing the fact that the expectancy rates for relatives of schizophrenics are much higher than for the general population. Also Vorster (1960) found 17 per cent incidence of schizophrenia in two-egg twins, as compared with 70 per cent of incidence in one-egg twins.

Diverse Points of View

Böök (1960) and Slater (1953, 1958) strongly criticized Kallmann's hypothesis of recessive heredity. They pointed out that, since the corrected risk figures for schizophrenia "do not differ to a significant degree between parents, siblings, and children with one or no affected parent" (Böök, 1960, p. 29), the hypothesis becomes untenable. Furthermore Gregory (1960) noted that the incidence of schizophrenia among various kinds of relatives follows neither a simple dominant nor a simple recessive pattern.

Böök hypothesized that schizophrenia could be caused by gene difference expressed in homozygotes in a recessive and occasionally in heterozygotes in a dominant fashion. The basis for this hypothesis is the concept of "reduced penetrance," i.e., the presence of a genetic factor does not necessarily affect the individual carrying it. Böök admitted (1960, p. 31) that the applicability of the concept of penetrance to humans has been questioned; however, this was the only way to reconcile conflicting statistical data. Garrone (1962) applied the penetrance hypothesis to a study of the population of schizophrenics in Geneva, and his findings showed that schizophrenia is inherited according to a simple recessive mode with 67 per cent of homozygous penetrance, thus arriving at practically the same results as Kallmann.

Loretta Bender (1956) also favors a genetic theory of schizophrenia. She proposed the hypothesis that schizophrenia is a process of dysmaturation and lag in development at the embryonic level which is hypothetically determined by genetic factors. The schizophrenic child is born with a kind of primitive *plasticity*. The entire neurological system of the child shows evidence of an organic lag in development. The infant's sleep, respiration, blood circulation, muscular tone, and metabolic processes are disturbed. The trauma caused by birth activates certain defense mechanisms which develop into the typical behavior patterns of schizophrenia. Thus

Bender sees in schizophrenia a sort of *encephalopathy* (1942, 1947a, 1947b, 1953, 1956, 1968).

Several research workers have supported Bender's hypothesis. Fish (1959) reported that a child diagnosed as schizophrenic at the age of five may have shown neurological and physiological disturbances as early as one month of age. Goldfarb (1961), however, found no significant differences in physical appearance between normal and schizophrenic children, and Eisenberg (1957) questioned the anatomical evidence of Bender's theory of encephalopathy. On the other hand, Bergman and Escalona (1949) reported unusual sensitivity in infants who were later diagnosed as psychotic. Their information, however, is based on parental observation, and there is no evidence demonstrating whether these sensitivities are inherited or acquired.

Roth (1957) stated that "no simple genetic hypothesis accords with all the facts." Rosenthal is basically in favor of a genetic interpretation of schizophrenia but admits that the question of what is actually inherited will remain unclear "until the specific metabolic error can be located or the specific patterns of influence defined or established" (1960).

D. Jackson (1960) examined the literature pertaining to genetics in schizophrenia and found that schizophrenia does not seem to follow the rules of dominant heredity. Furthermore, if schizophrenia were a product of recessive heredity, as Kallmann maintains, the rate of expectancy for monozygotic twins and for children of two schizophrenic parents would be 100 per cent. Yet Kallmann's rates are definitely lower. Kallmann's explanation that severe schizophrenics have no children is correct, but this does not prove that the nonexisting children of severe schizophrenics would necessarily be schizophrenic.

Karlsson introduced a two-factor genetic theory of schizophrenia. In his book *The Biologic Basis of Schizophrenia* (1966), Karlsson proposed that schizophrenia is caused by two major genes, one of them being dominant, the other recessive. Karlsson compared 24 true siblings with 28 foster home siblings of schizophrenic children who were adopted in their first year of life. Six of the biological siblings and none of the foster siblings developed schizophrenia. Karlsson's data seemingly offered a solid support for geneticity in childhood schizophrenia, if not for the loose use of the term schizophrenia in his studies. Karlsson, for instance, included manic-depressive psychosis in schizophrenia. Furthermore Karlsson assumed that the risk of schizophrenia in children who have two schizophrenic parents should be 68 per cent. Rosenthal (1966), however, proved that it cannot be higher than 38 per cent. Moreover, Rosenthal pointed out the possibility of intrauterine rather than genetic import of mother's schizophrenia on her schizophrenic offspring.

Money and Hirsch (1963), in a study of 784 female and 916 male mentally retarded cases, found three triple X and two triple XY; two of the cases were diagnosed as mentally retarded schizophrenic. The authors embarked upon a detailed pedigree study that proved that schizophrenia cannot be related to the X chromosome. In a recent summary of genetic studies Hurst (1970) wrote that "To date chromosomal anomalies have been demonstrated in only a very small minority of schizophrenic cases."

Critique of Twin Studies

Almost all studies in genetic aspects of schizophrenia point to the *possibility* of heredity, but they hardly prove it. The high concordance rates of incidence of schizophrenia in parents and children and in children and their siblings cannot serve as a proof of heredity, for these high correlations could be explained also by *intrafamilial interaction*.

The research concerning identical twins is the only true stronghold of genetic theories in schizophrenia. In data obtained by Kallmann, Slater, Garrone, and others are quite impressive, and seem to support the genetic theory of childhood schizophrenia. However, Jackson (1960) criticized the twin studies showing that practically all reported cases describe twins reared together and therefore cannot be used as a proof of heredity.

Also Rosenthal (1959, 1960, 1962) in surveys of twin studies noticed that almost all schizophrenic twins have been reared together, and this fact might have contributed to the high concordance. Moreover, the monozygotic fetal twins usually share a common maternal circulation, which may be disadvantageous to one of them and increase discordance in regard to various aspects of the illness. Twins are usually born prematurely and, therefore, constitute a deviant sample. Rosenthal, analyzing Slater's data, hypothesized that in paranoid schizophrenia in twins the genetic factor is minimal or absent, while it is considerable in catatonic twins. However, the study by Kringlen (1964) failed to corroborate Rosenthal's hypothesis.

Lidz et al. (1962) emphasized the peculiar symbiotic relationship that develops between a pair of monozygotic twins. Within the framework of the morbid intrafamilial situation, one of the twins usually assumes the dominating role. When one of them becomes schizophrenic, the other one suffers a psychotic breakdown also.

Kringlen (1966) in a study of 174 pairs of twins obtained results contradictory to Kallmann's data. The concordance data reported by Kringlen are much lower than Kallmann's, as is shown in Table 2.

Including schizophrenotype psychoses, Kringlen obtained somewhat higher concordance rates, namely 38 per cent for monozygotic twins and 14 per cent for dizygotic twins of the same sex, still much lower than Kallmann's data. "My general conclusion," Kringlen wrote, "was that the earlier studies (Kallmann, Slater, and others) probably contained many sources of error, the most important of which resided in the sampling techniques that gave results in which the genetic factor was overestimated" (1966, p. 183).

Apparently, the twin research has so far failed to prove heredity in childhood schizophrenia.

Diagnostic Categories

Some research workers suggested subdividing schizophrenia into two or more separate categories, one organic and the other sociopsychogenic. Bellak, for instance, suggested a multiple factor theory of schizophrenia (1949, 1958), and scores of research workers have offered a variety of theories, some of which will be described later on.

TABLE 2

	Number of Pairs	Concordant	Discordant	Per cent Concordant
Monozygotics	40	12	28	30
Dizygotics, same sex	74	4	70	5
Dizygotics, opposite sex	60	4	56	7

The apparent and extreme discrepancies make one wonder whether all the cases reported by various research workers belong to the study of schizophrenia. Karlsson (1966), as mentioned above, included manic-depressives as a subclass of schizophrenia; Bender (1959) included psychopathic behavior in schizophrenia. In view of an apparent lack of precision in diagnostic categories and differential diagnostic methods, one cannot avoid ambiguity in results of research.

As long as research workers do not operate with clearcut diagnostic categories, the etiological controversies cannot be solved. For instance, Rimland (1964) tried to prove that infantile autism is a distinct organic clinical entity. One cannot exclude the possibility that certain autistic symptoms are genosomatogenic (organic), but as will be explained later in this chapter and in Chapter 3, *certain* schizophrenic children develop autistic symptoms without any indication of organicity. Thus, Chapter 3 does not describe every possible sign of autism but rather the *autistic syndrome* of childhood schizophrenia.

The possibility of genetic origins of childhood schizophrenia remains a controversial issue. The loose diagnostic categories are a formidable obstacle, and as long as this lack of clarity prevails, research workers will contradict each other and sometimes contradict themselves (more about this problem in Chapter 6). One must, therefore, conclude that "heredity in schizophrenia is far from being a closed issue, and intensive research in the genetics of schizophrenia is being conducted at the present time in several scientific centers the world over." (Wolman, 1965c, p, 981.)

3. NEUROLOGICAL AND BIOCHEMICAL FACTORS

Intrauterine Life

Several research workers have observed a variety of organic symptoms in schizophrenic children. Some schizophrenic children suffer diarrhea, vomiting, and colic from their earliest days. Many of them rock, bang their heads, and develop peculiar motor discordinations apparent to any visitor to a children's ward in a mental hospital. It is not therefore surprising that serious neurological and biochemical research has been conducted aiming at the discovery of the origins of childhood schizophrenia.

Some research workers stress intrauterine rather than genetic factors. Sontag (1960) emphasized the importance of prenatal nutrition, oxygen supply, and the maternal fetal endocrine system. Pollin et al. (1965) traced the dissimilarities in identical twins to intrauterine experiences, "notably local anatomical peculiarities of the site of implantation within the uterus with subsequent unequal crowding; lateral inversion; and circulatory differences," and also to the differential impact of labor and delivery. Rosenthal (as mentioned before) stressed the import of prenatal life.

Postnatal Factors

Several workers point to early postnatal noxious factors. For instance Anderson (1952) believed that schizophrenia is often a result of anoxia in early childhood that may cause specific brain deficit in the child. This brain deficit might be any degree from minimal to severe and most likely affects the associational pathways of the superficial layers of the cortex. The deficit is believed to be in the adrenal system. Several factors can cause this deficit, among them measles, pneumonia, mother's shock at birth, mother's uterine hemorrhage at the end of pregnancy, or the infant's whooping cough, head injury, etc.

Sackler et al. (1952) observed that childhood schizophrenia is characterized by uneven intellectual, emotional, motor, and social development. According to these authors, such a regression or retardation is associated with neurological, physiological, and psychological factors. They believe that when schizophrenia occurs before the age of four it is probably a product of postnatal or prenatal neuroendocrine disturbances, especially maternal thyroid dysfunction. The higher incidence of childhood schizophrenia in males as compared with females seems to support their neuroendocine theory.

Postnatal factors may include endocrinopathy, also characteristic pallor, sexual precocity, gait disturbances, awkwardness in actions and plasticity, high blood glutamic acid and high adrenocortical concentration.

Eickhoff (1952) hypothesized that childhood schizophrenia, as an arrest in the development of abstract thought and emotional maturity at the infant or toddler level, is a result of a defect in neurological systems concerned with touch, pain, temperature, position, and vibration of senses or of faulty stimulation from outside or both.

Also Vorster (1960) assumed that schizophrenia is a product of both organic and sociopsychological factors. Brain damage may predispose to childhood schizophrenia, but if the intrafamilial emotional atmosphere is supportive, ego deficiency symptoms may not develop.

Biochemical Research

Several researchers (see Freeman's review of literature, 1958) have related schizophrenia to an alleged increase in cerebrospinal protein level, but no conclusive results have been obtained. Davidson (1960) and Hyden (1961) did not find any evidence with regard to the alleged role of RNA and protein in the etiology of schizophrenia. Other research workers, among them R. Gjessing (1938, p. 196), R. G. Hoskins (1946), Hoagland (1952), Reiss (1954), and others, believe hormonal disbalance to be the cause of schizophrenia. Yet these workers have not been able to agree as to whether it is thyroid or adrenalin or any other endocrine disorder that acts as the cause. M. Bleuler (1954), Freeman (1958), and others have stated, however, that there is no established connection between schizophrenia and endocrine factors.

In 1962 Friedhoof and Van Winkle identified 3,4-dimethoxyphenylethylamine in the urine of 15 out of 19 schizophrenics and none in the 14 controls. These findings have been confirmed by other research workers, among them Shulgin et al. (1967), von Studnitz (1965), Williams (1966), and others. However, Fourbye et al. (1966) failed to find this component in the urine of schizophrenic children.

Hendrickson believes that schizophrenia is "an organic abnormality of the nervous system, really a complex and subtle type of neurological disorder" (1952, p. 10). Yet even the most detailed research in brain activity (Davidson, 1960; Hyden, 1961) has not reached the point where one could conclusively state that schizophrenic behavior *is* caused by a smaller amount of RNA in the ganglion cells, as compared with normal controls.

As previously mentioned, Bender believes that organic determinants are the cause of schizophrenia. She stated that "childhood schizophrenia involves a maturational lag at the embryonic level. . . characterized by a primitive plasticity in all areas from which subsequent behavior results" (Bender, 1956, p. 499). Similar views have been expressed by A. M. Freedman (1954).

Kety expressed serious doubts as to whether "a generalized defect in energy metabolism . . . could be responsible for highly specialized features of schizophrenia" (1960) and Böök (1960, p. 32) found that the data on toxicity was very controversial. Richter (1957), on the basis of his own work and on that of others including R. Fisher, H. H. De Jong, H. Hoagland, and I. Munkvael, concluded that no evidence had been found as indication of free amino or any specific toxic compounds or abnormal metabolites in the blood of schizophrenics.

Heath (1960) proposed that "schizophrenia is a disease characterized by alterations in the metabolic pathways for the breakdown of certain endogenously occurring compounds" (p. 146). The presence of taraxein in the blood stream causes a toxic compound that alters the activities of certain parts of the brain and results in schizophrenic behavior.

Heath and associates reported on several occasions that a psychosis-inducing gamma globulin fraction in the sera of schizophrenic patients designated *taraxein,* was demonstrable by passive transfer in volunteer nonpsychotic recipients and in rhesus monkeys. In a paper published in 1968 Heath and Krupp stated that "the presence of taraxein in the sera of schizophrenic patients is specifically related to acute psychotic episodes and that serum fractions of patients with psychotic diseases other than schizophrenia produced negative results."

However, Heath's experimental results could not be consistently replicated in other laboratories. His theoretical conclusions based on his own observations are therefore open to doubt.

Kety reported (1960) that injection of taraxein caused symptoms resembling schizophrenia, but that there is no evidence that taraxein causes schizophrenia. Furthermore, there is no evidence supporting the amino acid metabolism hypothesis. "The chromatographic search for supportive evidence is interesting and valuable," wrote Kety, but "the preliminary indications of differences that are characteristic of even a segment of the disease rather than artifactual or incidental has not yet been obtained" (1960, p. 127). For instance, the presence of phenolic acids in the urine of schizophrenics has been, according to the study of T. D. Mann and E. H. Lambrosse, "better correlated with the ingestion of this beverage [coffee] than with schizophrenia" (Kety, 1960). Kline (1958) pointed out that the alleged link between biochemical aberrations and psychosis is often a product of the peculiar food intake of institutionalized patients.

Several research workers experimented with injecting schizophrenic serum into animals and human subjects. Walaszek (1960) injected schizophrenic serum into rabbits. The hypothalamic adrenalin level rose to three to five times the normal level in a period of four to eight days. Bishop (1963) found that the injection of schizophrenic serum into rats considerably affected learning and retention processes. German (1963) found significant differences in reaction of rats to the injection of human normal and schizophrenic serum. However, a comparative study of blood serum of schizophrenic and nonschizophrenic children failed to discover significant differences concerning optical density and slope and lag time (Aprison, 1958).

Wooley's hypothesis (1958) with regard to the role played by the serotonin enzyme has been tested in the so-called "model psychosis." Yet Kety (1960), Szara (1958), and others report failure to find significant differences between normal controls and schizophrenics.

Reviews of research by Freeman (1958), Overholser and Werkman (1958), and Werkman (1959), and Kety (1960) did not disclose any clearly determined causal relationships between biochemical factors and schizophrenia.

Neurological Studies

More recent studies seem to focus on neurological determinants of schizophrenia, pointing to the interaction between these determinants and sociogenic factors. Neurological deficiencies are believed to serve as predisposing factors, and the child's interaction with the environment serve as precipitatory factors.

As early as 1949, Bergman and Escalona stated that children who show uneven development, and who eventually manifest psychotic disorganization, are characterized from a very early age by extreme sensitivity to various types of stimuli. They suggest that in these children there is a defect in the organic or neurophysiological barrier against these stimuli, and that the aberrant behavior of such children is an attempt to protect themselves against overpowering stimuli.

Pasamanick and Knobloch (1963), after a study of the literature regarding early feeding problems and the eventual development of schizophrenia, reported that it may be erroneous to correlate these problems with maternal rejection, as many writers have. They state that one of the most prominent causes of difficulty in nursing is due to *brain injury* in the child. Therefore, they suggest that a child with some sort of mild physical abnormality will exhibit pathological behavior such as refusal to suckle, which in turn may cause the mother to become anxious and even rejecting. The child's disability and the reaction to it on the part of the mother may eventually result in childhood schizophrenia or autism. Therefore Pasamanick and Knobloch state that it would be "advisable, at this time, to reconsider both the etiology and diagnosis of much of 'childhood schizophrenia' or 'infantile autism,' and possibly assign these cases to relevant chronic brain syndromes" (p. 76).

Also Leonberg and Bok (1967) wrote that, although no consistent anatomic-pathologic derangement of the central nervous system was found in schizophrenic children, research, "seems to indicate an organic basis for this disease" and "the interaction of organic and psychogenic factors may produce childhood schizophrenia."

As a result of a study of prenatal and perinatal factors in childhood schizophrenia, Taft and Goldfarb (1964) reported that "symptoms of childhood psychosis are expressions of adaptation to a diversity of elements, and that, in addition, brain damage can in itself be a primary causative agent for the ego deficits of some children in the constellation of children designated by the label of childhood schizophrenic" (*ibid.*, p. 32). In their study they found that a number of children diagnosed as schizophrenic had been traumatized and neurologically impaired in the course of the reproductive process. Taft and Goldfarb further add that "The cerebral dysfunction restricts the child's adaptive competence; the direct expressions of cerebral dysfunction stimulate responses from his parents; and these parental responses in turn became stimuli which reinforce behavior in the child which we term "schizophrenic" (*ibid.*, p. 42).

Gittelman and Birch (1967) made a similar study, and their findings support those of Taft and Goldfarb. Yet they feel that their data point to a theory proposing a continuum of psychogenicity interrelated with organismic factors. They state that psychotic children possess primary disorders of the sensory and response systems which predispose the child to abnormal patternings of organism-environmental interactions and which affect the totality of perceptual, cognitive, and interpersonal experiences which are vital to psychological growth.

Ornitz and Ritvo (1968) believe that there is a single, psychological process which is common to early infantile autism, certain cases of childhood schizophrenia, the atypical child, symbiotic psychosis and children with unusual sensitivities. While the symptoms of all these disorders include disturbances of perception, mobility, relatedness, language, and developmental rate, according to Ornitz and Ritvo perceptual disturbance is fundamental to the disorders and is evidenced by a very early failure to distinguish between self and the environment and the inability to imitate, and to modulate sensory input. These writers propose that schizophrenic children are unable to maintain perceptual constancy, due "to an underlying failure of homeostatic regulation with the central nervous system so that environmental stimulations are either not adequately modulated or are unevenly amplified" (*ibid.*, p. 88). Furthermore, the child's various symptoms are merely a result of this "pathophysiology" and are often the result of the child's attempt to adjust to the "pathophysiology."

Summarizing organic studies in etiology of childhood schizophrenia, Kanner wrote (1960):

> Much etiologic research has been directed towards endogenous factors. German and Dutch neuropathologists have combed the brain for indications of organic involvement; they were not successful in their efforts. Electroencephalographic studies have yielded no uniform pattern. Evidence of endocrine dysfunctions is scattered and, when present, does not answer unequivocally the question of cause and effect relationship. . . . Statistical studies have shown a greater prevalence of mental illness in the families of schizophrenics than in the average population. . . . The idea of heredity as chromosomal doom has been challenged of late by the consideration that psychotic parents, even when not acutely disturbed, bring severe conflicts to the relationship with their children; do these conflicts and their impact which can be studied concretely, mean less than the presence of psychotic ancestors which impresses one mainly because of the relative frequency? . . . Even from a purely statistical point of view, the correlation of childhood schizophrenia with parental attitudes is far higher and more consistent than its correlation with heredity, configuration of the body, metabolic disorders or any other factor. . . .

Sociopsychosomatic Theory

No one can deny the fact that schizophrenia affects the organism and that schizophrenic children display a variety of somatic symptoms. The question is of *causal* order, namely, is schizophrenia a somatopsychosocial or a sociopsychosomatic disorder? (Wolman, 1967).

There have been a variety of answers to this question. For instance Osmond and Hoffer (1966) maintain that their "adrenochrome metabolite theory provides a means by which a genetic mechanism could produce the physiological, biochemical and clinical peculiarities found in schizophrenia. These result in perceptual and affective changes which determine the extensive psychosocial consequences." However, so far biochemical and neurological studies have failed to adduce adequate causal evidence and, quite often, the data obtained by various research workers contradict each other. Moreover, Richter (1957) in a review of diversified organic research concluded that "it is always difficult to distinguish between cause and effect" (1957, p. 68).

A great part of research that points to the etiologic organicity of schizophrenia has been conducted on chronic schizophrenics, most of them in their middle or old age. For instance, Brambilla et al. (1967) in a study of 72 chronic schizophrenics aged 14-53 found that endocrine glands are impaired, and that the severity of the glandular impairment corresponds to the severity and the age of onset of the disorder. Most striking pathology was found in hebephrenics with onset at puberty. The results obtained with schizophrenics whose manifest disorder was recent were rather negative. Especially striking are the negative results obtained by Aprison and Drew (1958) and Fourbye et al. (1966) in regard to children (see above). These results indicate that *biochemical symptoms follow psychological* (behavioral) symptoms, suggesting that in schizophrenia the psychological changes are the *cause* and not the results of somatic changes.

For instance, a study by Gottlieb and associates of carbohydrate metabolism in schizophrenia offers further support to the sociopsychosomatic theory. Becket et al. (1963) found that premorbid social isolation and diminished heterosexual drive were related to biochemical abnormalities." Specifically the mother of the schizophrenic patient was a "shielding, protecting person who did not allow her son to experience the ordinary stimulation and challenges of childhood. . . . A hypothesis is presented suggesting that a certain amount of stimulation in early life is necessary for the proper maturation of the energy-producing metabolic system."

Practically all empirical findings speak in favor of such a causal chain. There is no doubt that *many* (but not all) adult schizophrenics and some children with severe cases of schizophrenia develop somatic symptoms. There is little evidence that schizophrenic behavior is a result of these biochemical afflictions, for many individuals with metabolic troubles ascribed to schizophrenia never become schizophrenic. There is, however, a substantial, though by no means, conclusive evidence that *schizophrenia can produce all these biochemical disorders.*

There is no doubt that emotional stress may cause biochemical changes, especially in the adrenocortical and thyroid systems, as well as in the production of epinephrine and norepinephrine. These changes are not a cause but an *effect* of emotional stress.

Freud (1924, 1927, 1949), Fenichel (1945), and most psychoanalysts believe that schizophrenia is a narcissistic disorder. Accordingly, "many schizophrenics begin characteristic hypochondriacal sensations. The beginning of the schizophrenic process is a regression to narcissism. This brings with it an increase in the 'libido tonus' of the body (either of the whole body, or depending on the individual history, of certain organs) and this increase makes itself felt in the form of the hypochondriacal sensations" (Fenichel, 1945, p. 418).

This theory does not, however, sound too convincing, for narcissistic individuals usually take good care of themselves. But when someone cares so much for others as to neglect oneself, his *hypocathected* body may react with symptom formation. Practically all the schizophrenics I have ever seen suffered from low vitality and lack of energy, and a great many of them suffered a variety of respiratory diseases and caught frequent colds. Skin diseases usually developed in their least cathected organs. A girl who doubted her manual dexterity had a severe skin rash on her hands; another, who believed she was ugly, had a facial rash; still another, who doubted her femininity, had a skin rash on her pubic area. The theory of self-hypocathexis in schizophrenia (introduced by Federn, 1952), explains the decline in sensitivity to pain, and the generally lowered tonus and passivity in schizophrenia. The schizophrenic tendency for self-mutilation is well explained by the theory of *decline* in self-cathexis.

The hypothesis of somatic symptoms resulting from hypocathexis of bodily organs completes the *sociopsychosomatic* theory. My observations have led me to believe that noxious *environmental* (social) factors cause an imbalance in *interindividual cathexes*. This imbalance produces a severe disbalance in the *intraindividual* cathexes of libido and destrudo; this, in turn, introduces a disorder in the personality structure (psychological factors). The personality disorder causes somatic changes, either through a transformation of deficiency in mental energy into organic deficiencies or through the process of conditioning (Wolman, 1966, 1967).

Research in conditioning reported by Buck et al. (1950), Bykov (1957), Gantt (1958), Hamburg (1958), Ivanov-Smolensky (1954), Lynn (1963), Malis (1961), Mednick (1958), and others distinctly points to such a possibility. Psychologically induced changes in heartbeat, rate of metabolism, circulation of blood, or respiration are not limited to Charcot's hysterics. They are common to all human beings, including schizophrenics, and can be produced by conditioning or cathexis or both. In schizophrenia these processes follow the direction of a "downward adjustment."

Impulses coming from the cortex may inhibit the activity of an organ. Overworked cortical centers may interfere with the work of other organs. New "connections" are being formed, and the inner organs become conditioned to react in an unusual way, even if this is detrimental to the survival of the organism. This influence seems to be *inhibitory,* and reduces the vitality of schizophrenics. "It may be assumed" wrote Bykov (1957, p. 140) "that in acting on the functioning cells of the salivary glands, the nervous impulses from the cortex along the efferent nerves reduce the excitation of the salivary glands to a minimum. . . . A weak excitation on reaching a slightly functioning gland increased its activity, whereas a strong excitation inhibited it."

Also the magnitude of the general metabolism can be changed through conditioning by word signals. The sound of metronome and the command, "Get ready for the experiment," caused in experimental subjects a marked increase in oxygen consumption and pulmonary ventilation. In one experiment, "a man who remained quietly lying on a couch showed an increase in metabolism when suggested that he had just completed some very hard muscular work" (Bykov, 1957, p. 179). In another experiment the rate of metabolism went up in a subject who imagined that he was working.

In terms of the sociopsychosomatic theory, schizophrenia is an impoverishment of one's own resources and a struggle for survival, caused by a morbid hypervectorialism. This state of mind may correspond to a cerebrospinal hypertension, for *sociopsychological stimuli cause somatic changes.*

Analgesias are another example of the same issue. E. Bleuler wrote in 1911: "Even in well oriented patients one may often observe the presence of a complete *analgesia* which includes the deeper parts of the body as well as the skin. The patients intentionally or unintentionally incur quite serious injuries, pluck out an eye, sit down on a hot stove and receive severe gluteal burns," etc. (E. Bleuler, 1950, p. 57).

Analgesias can be produced by conditioning (Bykov, 1957, p. 342) and/or by a low self-cathexis. The decline in self-cathexis makes the schizophrenic less capable of loving and protecting himself, but in face of real danger, schizophrenics may display a self-defensive reaction. Severely deteriorated cases, however, with their lowest sensitivity to pain, may fall victim to any danger.

Severely deteriorated schizophrenics appear insensitive when the flame of a candle is passed rapidly over the skin. They may sit near the radiator and, if they are not moved, they may continue to stay there even when, as a result of close contact, they are burned. They "seem to have lost the sensation of taste. When they are given bitter radishes or teaspoons of sugar, salt, pepper or quinine, they do not show any pleasant or unpleasant reaction" (Arieti, 1955, pp. 373-374).

This is the *schizophrenic paradox:* real life is sacrificed for a pseudo protection of life. The schizophrenic feels he has to give away his life to protect those upon whom his survival depends. His lavish hypercathexis of his "protectors" leads to his own impoverishment and eventual death (Wolman, 1966).

A radical decline in pain sensation, whether interpreted by conditioning or lack of self-cathexis, destroys the individual's ability to protect his own life.

Arieti (1955, p. 392) believes that the following four changes usually take place in the cardiovascular system of schizophrenics, namely, (1) a decrease in the size of the heart, (2) decrease in the volume of blood flow, (3) decrease in systematic blood pressure, and (4) an exaggerated tendency to vasoconstriction and resulting diminished blood supply. Arieti believes that all these are psychosomatic products of schizophrenia.

Several research workers (Hoskins, 1946) implied that schizo-phrenics suffer from a defect in their vasomotor systems or in nerve control apparatus of this system, located in the hypothalamus. Also cyanosis or the blueing of hands and feet caused by venous stasis is frequently observed in schizophrenics. This symptom has been often interpreted as a constriction of the small arterioles of the skin. Doust (1952) found a significant degree of anoxemia in simple, catatonic, and hebephrenic schizophrenics. The existence of a cerebral anoxe-mia could not be proved. The passive behavior of schizophrenics may prevent dissipation of heat. Furthermore, the bizarre posture of cata-tonics "activate antigravity vasoconstrictor mechanisms. Without these mechanisms, edema due to blood stasis would be very frequent" (Arieti, 1955, p. 395). The regulation of heat exchange in the hu-man body is of particular interest in the study of schizophrenia. My own patients have chronically complained in winter about inade-quate heat; it seems that schizophrenics are more sensitive to cold. Buck et al. (1950) found the rectal temperature of schizophrenics significantly lower than that of normal subjects.

Schizophrenic regression is apparently a process that starts from social relations, affects the personality, and may ultimately lead to a physical decline also.

4. SOCIOCULTURAL DETERMINANTS

Hollingshead and Redlich (1958) found in their Yale study that severity of mental disorder was inversely related to socioeconomic class, and the prevalent rate of schizophrenia in the lowest class was eight times higher than in the highest socioeconomic class. Hare (1955) in England also found a positive correlation between schizo-phrenia and exceedingly low socioeconomic status. Goldhamer (1949), however, questioned the reliability of the Hollingshead and Redlich study because of the small number of cases.

Stein (1957, quoted by Wolman, 1965c), in her study of mental disorders in London, found higher incidence of schizophrenia in two boroughs; while there was a lower rate of schizophrenia in the more wealthy borough, a higher rate was found in the lowest economic class of each borough.

Although the incidence of schizophrenia seems to be highest in the lowest socioeconomic class, the fathers of schizophrenics represent all socioeconomic classes. The low socioeconomic status of schizo-phrenics may therefore not be a cause but rather a result of schizo-phrenia. Kanner's early study (1943) is a case in point, for Kanner found that most parents of schizophrenic children belong to the middle and upper social class.

Apparently schizophrenia is not related to socioeconomic status. Families of wealthy schizophrenics, as well as families of other wealthy patients, seek help from private practitioners, while schizo-phrenics from low income classes are most frequently committed to mental institutions (Wolman, 1966).

Studies of the relationship between schizophrenia and urbanization and social mobility (Faris and Dunham, 1939) suggest that there is some connection between these factors. However, Freedman's find-ings (1950) of the relationship between high mobility and high hos-pital admission rates of schizophrenics did not support Fairs' and Dunham's hypothesis.

In a review of the literature, Lemkau and Crocetti concluded that "there is a great deal of evidence justifying the speculation that there is an etiological relationship between schizophrenia and urbanization. However, the nature of the relationship or even its unchallenged existence has not yet been completely demonstrated" (1958, p. 73).

Von Brauchitsch and Kirk (1967), found that childhood schizo-phrenia was more frequently discovered in upper socioeconomic classes; it was least frequent in children from broken homes, hard-core multiproblem families, and families with overt mental illness among the parents. Furthermore, the prognosis of schizophrenia in the upper classes is less favorable and most closely resembles adult forms of psychoses, while children in the lower classes seem to lapse in and out of schizophrenic behavior. They state that "It is possible that certain characteristic features of the disease [i.e., autistic and symbiotic symptoms and poor prognosis] are related to parental atti-tudes and ultimately to social group pressure rather than to the dis-ease proper" (p. 400).

Migration is believed to be highly correlated with schizophrenia. Malzberg and Lee (1956) found that psychosis rates were twice as high for migrants as for nonmigrants, but it was not clearly evident that rates of schizophrenia were especially high. Yet studies by Øde-gaard (1932, 1945) and Wolman (1946, 1949) point to the conclusion that problems due to *acculturation* related to migration, but not migration as such, created emotional conflict. In most cases migration affects the socioeconomic status of fathers.

People migrate because they have not been successful in their homeland and expect a radical improvement in the new country. Apparently, migration often brings serious disappointments, or at least, temporary ones. Children attend school, learn the new language, and may adjust quickly. Parents, and especially the fathers as breadwinners, may find their skills inadequate, their earning capacity limited, and their foreign customs and language subject to ridicule. The fathers may remain "greenhorns" for a long time, and their adjustment hardships invoke lack of respect from the members of their own families. The above-mentioned studies (Wolman, 1946, 1949) point to a decline of paternal authority and distinct confusion of social status and roles in those migratory families that produced schizophrenic offspring (more about families in the next section of this chapter.)

Studies dealing with sociocultural and ethnic factors in etiology of schizophrenia have yielded rather inconsistent results, and conclusions related to a schizogenic influence of any particular ethnic group seen to be wholly unwarranted. In a review of sociocultural research on etiology of childhood schizophrenia, Sanua (1961) wrote that "generalization from these studies should be limited in scope. A lack of consistency in the findings can largely be attributed to a partial or total neglect of important variables." Linton (1956) in a study of a variety of cultural patterns also arrived at the conclusion that schizophrenia is not related to any particular culture.

5. FAMILY DYNAMICS

Apparently the etiology of childhood schizophrenia remains a controversial issue, for no theory has been able to muster conclusive evidence. There is, however, a growing body of empirical data in support of intrafamilial relationships as the main if not the sole cause of childhood schizophrenia.

However, even this hypothesis lacks final evidence, and research workers who stress family dynamics by no means agree with one another.

Parental Personalities

Several authors maintain that the parents of schizophrenics are either schizophrenics themselves or represent a variety of severe mental cases. However, observational and statistical studies do not bear out the hypothesis that the parents of schizophrenic children are necessarily schizophrenic themselves, nor that they form a clear-cut pathological group. Kanner (1943), Kanner and Eisenberg (1955), Despert (1951), Rank (1955), Nuffield (1954), Rosen (1953), and others found the parents of schizophrenics and especially the mothers, to be highly disturbed, narcissistic, cold, etc. Some writers have used the term "schizogenic mother," but there has been no agreement in regard to the personality traits that make a mother "schizogenic."

Furthermore, research workers failed to find any definite pathology in the parents of schizophrenics. Alanen (1958) found 10 per cent of the parents of schizophrenics to be disturbed and slightly over 5 per cent schizophrenic. I have found (Wolman, 1961, 1965a, 1966) about 40 per cent of fathers and 30 per cent of mothers of schizophrenics displaying a great variety of pathological conditions, but it was impossible to state that schizophrenia in offspring is caused by any peculiar mental type of parents.

Kanner (1960) believes that there is a typical, consistent pattern in the attitudes of the parents of schizophrenic children toward their children. According to Kanner, the parents of schizophrenic children are cold, intellectual, compulsive, detached, objective, and mechanical in their dealings with their children; he called them "refrigerator" parents. It seemed to him that these children's withdrawal was a turning from this situation to find comfort in being alone.

Kanner and Eisenberg, in a follow-up study of 105 cases, wrote the following about both parents: "The majority of parents. . . were cold, detached, humorless perfectionists" (1955). Arieti found that among the parents of schizophrenics there is a predominance of a "domineering, nagging and hostile mother, who gives the child no chance to assert himself, [who] is married to a dependent, weak man, too weak to help the child" (1955 p. 52).

Research workers at the James Jackson Putnam Center (Rank, 1949, 1955; Putnam, 1955; and others) believe that the most important etiological factors were related to "profound disturbance" in early parent-child relationship and traumatic events, especially separation from parents (Rank, 1955, p. 493). Rank points to a "fragmented ego" that is "the result of the infant's unsuccessful struggle to obtain vital satisfaction from his parents" (*ibid.*)

Rank's findings agree with Kanner's, that childhood schizophrenia is a result of impact of a narcissistic and immature mother who is not able to offer to the infant a favorable environment for the formation and differentiation of one's own ego and the establishment of the reality principle. Thus the withdrawal of schizophrenic children is seen as an escape from a world which is dangerous.

Kaufman et al. (1959) claim that the parents of schizophrenic children suffer *severe ego disturbances*. The parents ward off their anxiety, with which their defective ego cannot cope, by projecting the anxiety onto the child who as a result will become schizophrenic. Many disturbed parents actively interfere with the child's attempt to perceive reality and convey to the child their ideas of unreality and perceptual distortions.

The parents of schizophrenic children do not offer guidance and control. They fail to reinforce clear concepts of time and space because their own life is disorganized. They offer no reward or punishment, nor do they meet the child's needs for gratification. They communicate in a confusing manner and give conflicting instructions (Bateson et al., 1956; Goldfarb and Mintz, 1961; Wolman, 1957, 1966). "Regardless of the externals of their behavior, these parents all show a similar core disturbance. They express the fear that experiencing their inner tensions will lead to their own total destruction or annihilation." (Kaufman et al., 1960, p. 920.)

Kaufman et al. (1960) divided the parents of schizophrenic children into four separate categories, namely, the pseudo-neurotic, the somatic, the pseudo-delinquent, and the overtly psychotic. Pseudo-neurotic parents are frequently professionals who have achieved high ranks in their field. They utilize neurotic defenses to maintain the "rigid, stereotyped life situation," (p. 920) and often identify themselves with their schizophrenic child.

Somatic parents are usually skilled laborers, teachers, nurses, small businessmen, etc. They are perplexed by hypochondriac fears and experience frequent somatic disturbances.

Pseudo-delinquent parents are usually bartenders, armed service personnel, criminals, alcoholics, and transient laborers who externalize their psychotic anxieties through antisocial behavior.

Overtly psychotic parents are usually farmers, junk dealers, taxi-cab drivers, office clerks, house painters, etc. They experience delusions of grandeur, distortions of reality, and hallucinations.

Many workers have described the mothers of schizophrenic children as extremely immature, narcissistic individuals who possess narcissistic qualities and who are usually incapable of having mature emotional relationships.

Tietz divided the mothers of schizophrenic children into the three following types: (1) overly demanding, hostile, but superficially sweet and polite mothers, (2) docile, submissive mothers who eagerly and excessively cooperate, but who are perfectionists and who dominate others through a sense of dependence, and, (3) overly rejecting mothers. The schizophrenogenic mothers manipulate and exploit their child (Block et al., 1958).

Cheek (1964) studied mothers in 67 families with schizophrenic young adults. The mothers of schizophrenics proved to be cold and withdrawn in comparison with the mothers of normal young adults in 56 families. Gianascol (1963) did not find a consistent pathology in parents of schizophrenic children, but every parent manifested severe anxiety, ambivalence, and projections.

Waring and Ricks (1965) compared 50 schizophrenics to 50 controls. Their conclusions follow:

1. Seriously disturbed chronic schizophrenics are more likely than controls to have mothers who were themselves psychotic, schizoid, or borderline character disorders.

2. The so-called schizo- or schizophrenogenic mothers were found in all groups, but most of these mothers raised children who were not hospitalized; chronic schizophrenics have had the smallest number of these mothers.

3. Many mothers of discharged schizophrenic patients appeared to be depressed or have had prolonged periods of depression during the childhood of the patient.

4. The *severity* of the mother's disturbance was more predictive of schizophrenia in the child than the *type* of her disturbance.

The study conducted by Waring and Ricks (1965) indicates that psychotic and schizoid fathers were found among 40 per cent of the patients, 17 per cent of the discharged, and 10 per cent of the controls. Impulsive character disorders and neurotic adjustments within the normal range, were more frequent among the fathers of the controls than among those of the schizophrenics. Reactive or characterlogic depression occurred as a symptom less frequently among the fathers in all groups than among the mothers.

Waring and Ricks concluded:

1. Most chronic schizophrenics come from prolonged symbiotic parent-child relationships. No emotionally healthy child could have developed within such an environment.

2. Chaotic family relationships occurred less frequently among the schizophrenic group than among the controls.

3. Discharged schizophrenics came from families which expelled the child. The relatively better prognosis for children from such families could be explained by the opportunity that expulsion from the morbid family offered for the formation of healthier relationships elsewhere.

4. No emotionally healthy families produced children who became schizophrenics.

The type of family environment most productive of chronic schizophrenics was a prolonged symbiotic union between a parent and the preschizophrenic child.

Some authors maintain that the fathers of schizophrenic children are often more disturbed than the mothers and that many of them show schizoid patterns of behavior. Both parents fail to present themselves to their child in a consistent, clearly defined behavioral pattern (Esman et al., 1959).

According to Klebanoff (1959) the problem of etiology of childhood schizophrenia is represented by two main hypotheses, namely: (1) the *biogenic* hypothesis, which maintains that there is as yet an undiscovered organic reason for the child's symptoms, the mother's pathological attitudes to the child being a *result* of the stress of trying to deal with the disordered child; (2) the *psychogenic* hypothesis, which holds that the impact on the child of the mother's pathological attitudes toward child rearing and the family brings about a schizophrenic reaction.

Szurek (1956) found that, in all instances in which a child was diagnosed as schizophrenic, both parents were found to have suffered severe intrapsychic conflicts prior to the development of the child's disorder. Szurek states that the psychotic child's disorder represents his identification with and rebellion against each of the parent's disorders, while the healthy aspects of the child seem to be correlated with his integrative experiences with his parents. Furthermore the child's symptoms are often a caricature of what he sees in his parents.

My detailed case studies, which included 101 adult schizophrenics and 59 children and adolescents, are rather inconclusive (Wolman, 1933, 1936, 1957, 1965c, 1966). The parents of schizophrenics display a variety of pathological personality types, but no one can be sure that they would have produced schizophrenic children if each had married another person. An adequately controlled study should have checked the same or carefully matched pathological types in a different family setting, which is not easily done. At the present time there is no conclusive evidence that certain pathological parents cause schizophrenia in their children, but there is evidence that childhood schizophrenia is caused by a peculiar intrafamilial interaction.

Interactional Patterns

Several research workers studying the parents of schizophrenic children have arrived independently at the conclusion that the particular *interactional* patterns are of greater etiological significance than the personality characteristics of the parents. On my first job as clinical psychologist in the Centos Institute I noticed peculiar interparental strife amongst parents of schizophrenic children. Practically all parents I interviewed expressed a thinly veiled hostility to each other and competition for the child's love concealed under the disguise of a self-sacrificing love for their child (Wolman, 1933, 1936, 1943).

Several other workers have arrived at similar conclusions (Arieti, 1955; Gerard and Siegel, 1950; Hill, 1955; Kohn and Clausen, 1956; and others). A vivid description of the experiences of Dr. W. Elgin, is quoted by Hill (1955, p. 107): who was in charge of admissions to a psychiatric ward,

For many years Dr. Elgin, in the process of admitting patients, observed the enactment of a scene which assumed diagnostic significance. His office arrangement permitted relatives a choice of three seats, one opposite his desk, one at the end of it quite near him, and one several feet away. He observed that, when the mother and father of the patient appeared together to arrange admission, there occurred something of significance. If mother sat in one of the two chairs at his desk, and father sat off in a corner, it usually followed that mother took over the discussion, did the talking, made the arrangements, and even read the fine print on the contract. Father, meanwhile, looked unhappy and was silent save for an occasional abortive effort to modify certain of the mother's statements. When this was the course of the admission interview, he came to know that the odds were that the patient would be schizophrenic. There is an interesting addendum. In a later interview father, appearing alone, was often very aggressive in his criticism and his demands and accusations. However, it could often be demonstrated that his belligerence was that of a very unwilling agent of his wife.

It seems that research workers belonging to different schools of thought and using a variety of methods have come to an almost unanimous conclusion that schizophrenia is a result of faulty social relations in childhood. It is as if one could say that *schizophrenia is produced by mismanagement of men (children) by men (parents)*.

Behrens and Goldfarb (1958) found that most homes of schizophrenic children are physically deteriorated, uncared for, and overcrowded and are characterized by the absence of interest and pride in children by parents. A lack of spontaneity and pleasure is noticeable. An *isolation between mother and father* or between one of them and the child exists, and there is a general *lack of communication*. Interaction on a verbal level takes the form of malicious teasing and lack of affective content. The parents in many cases are immature in relation to each other as well as toward others. Many homes are also characterized by an atmosphere of confusion, continuous feud, or overt tug-of-war (Lidz et al., 1957, 1958, 1960).

In normal families the social status and role of each parent is more or less defined. The father supports the family and determines its social status and prestige, and the mother's main task is the responsibility for the inner works of the family. Each parent must also support his or her spouse through his or her power and emotional values.

In many families, both spouses are concerned with their own personality difficulties, which may or may not have been caused by the marital relationship. In either case, the marital relationship increases these difficulties. Neither spouse gains emotional support from the other spouse and usually recurrent threats of separation occur. There is little, if any, sharing of problems or satisfactions. Each spouse ignores the needs of his or her spouse, and it is very common for each parent to compete for the children's affection (Lidz et al., 1957).

In such a family, the father very often becomes an outsider or a secondary figure in the house as a result of his own behavior or the attitude of his wife toward him. The mother, on the other hand, is concerned with her household duties, but this excludes a relationship with her children. Her cold, rigid, and/or indulgent attitude towards her children antagonizes her husband. It becomes quite clear to the child who becomes schizophrenic that each spouse does not care for the other, and that he is required to supply to the frustrated parents the warmth that they cannot obtain from each other. Thus Fleck, summarizing the research work conducted by Lidz and his associates and their intensive study of schizogenic families arrived at the following conclusion (Fleck et al., 1959, p. 335):

We realized, soon, that the intrapsychic disturbances of the mothers were not nearly as relevant to what happened to one or more children in the family (especially to the child who became schizophrenic), as was the fact that these women were paired with husbands who would either acquiesce to the many irrational and bizarre notions of how the family should be run or who would constantly battle with and undermine an already anxious and insecure mother.

Schizogenic Families

In normal families, parents are perceived by their children as strong and friendly adults who relate to each other in a *mutual,* give-and-take manner, and have a *vectorial,* giving attitude toward the child, irrespective of what the child may be or do. Parental love is unconditional; the smaller and weaker the child, the more vectorial the parental attitude.

This vectorial, protecting attitude of the parents enables the instrumentally minded, narcissistic infant to progress toward higher levels of interindividual relations. For example, a child properly treated at the anal stage, graciously accepts toilet training with its demand of giving something away. The growing child "generalizes," this give-and-take or mutual acceptance attitude and gradually learns reciprocity in relations with his peers. This social development, brought about by both maturation and learning processes, helps the child to grow to a point where he will be able to assume a future vectorial attitude toward his children. The child who has had a normal family background develops into an adult capable of instrumental, mutual, and vectorial relationships.

Detailed case studies (Wolman, 1957, 1965a, 1966) show that it is not the "weak father and strong mother" who produce schizophrenia in their offspring. If this were so, *all* siblings of a schizophrenic would be schizophrenic. The empirical evidence is, however, to the contrary.

In all the cases of childhood schizophrenia I have seen in 30 years of practice, the intrafamilial relationship reflected practically the same pattern. Parents of schizophrenic children expect from each other the impossible, and they are, therefore, inevitably and painfully disappointed. They expect to be mothered and fathered by their husbands and wives respectively. They do not seek friendship and companionship in marriage, but hope to find a loving parent in their spouse.

A disappointed adult tends to discontinue an unsuccessful marriage and seek new relationships. A disappointed child pouts and cries, but stays home. Parents of schizophrenic children hate one another, complain, and quarrel, but divided they stand together (Lidz et al., 1957; Wolman, 1957, 1966) and hurt each other.

With the birth of the first child the situation becomes aggravated. Then the mothers make excessive demands of their husbands, requesting help in the household, attention and consideration, and an exaggerated support. Were their husbands more considerate, more supportive, and less demanding of support for themselves, these women could have possibly become adequate mothers. But since the men fail as husbands and fathers, the women became more domineering, more dictatorial, more demanding, and assume the tyrant-martyr attitude toward the child. They expect from the child what they fail to receive from their husbands, and entangle the child in a web of frustrated sexual needs and hurt emotions. In many instances the mothers of schizophrenic children avoid sexual relations with their husbands. Some of them use sex as a reward and punishment.

The husbands, rejected by their wives, maintain that the wives give all their love to the child. The wives, disappointed by the non-supporting husbands, turn marital relations either into a pseudo-respectful, cold, detached attitude to the husband ("kicking up"), an overt tug-of-war against him ("kicking down"), or an effort to throw him out of the home ("kicking out"). In any case the child who becomes schizophrenic becomes aware of the fact that father and mother hate each other. In cases where hostility has been overt, violent, and has led to physical fights, the greatest damage is caused to the child's personality and psychosis was severe.

Some mothers develop either a *parasitic-symbiotic* or a *hostile-protective* attitude toward the child. Whenever the mother is symbiotic, the child does not have much chance for development of his own personality. The situation is much worse when the mother, in a tug-of-war with the father, "protects" the child from the father and expresses overt hate to "his" child.

All mothers in schizophrenic families reduce the father's role to the role of an infant; some mothers fight the fathers and express disrespect for him in many ways. Some mothers demonstrate their "willingness to help" because without their help "the poor man" could not survive.

Most mothers censor the father's behavior, send him on errands, control his small expenses, and check his wallet and pockets. Some mothers tear their husbands down in the children's presence, criticize them publicly, ridicule and belittle their achievements, and rebuke and insult them daily (Wolman, 1961).

Most mothers mean well. Some explain that they have had no choice but to take over the role of father and mother. All of them somehow manage to force the husband out of his usual role as the leader and protector of the family. Certainly no woman could accomplish this without her husband's being the tacit or unprotesting accomplice; the fathers of schizophrenic patients, wittingly or unwittingly, help their wives in this morbid process.

Jane Slowman, the sixteen year old catatonic girl, was her daddy's "nice little girl." Mr. Slowman was a successful businessman married to an ambitious socialite. Mrs. Slowman came from a very wealthy family ruled high-handedly by a selfish, ruthless father. She was attracted to the easygoing, friendly Mr. Slowman, expecting him to compensate her for her unhappy childhood. Mrs. Slowman behaved as if she were a teenager, wishing her husband "to take care of her, to pamper her, and to shower her with gifts." Mr. Slowman has had similar hopes. He was the "forgotten child," and expected to be compensated in marriage for his sad childhood.

Obviously both Mr. and Mrs. Slowman wanted to be loved without being able to offer much in return. While they functioned reasonably well with peers and neighbors, they were unable to accept marriage in an adult way. They interacted with each other in a childish way, fighting for little privileges, complaining and accusing each other for being selfish.

When Jane was born, both parents felt more frustrated than ever. Mr. Slowman felt "left out" and "rejected" by his wife's preoccupation with the baby. Mrs. Slowman demanded more paternal care than ever, and felt gravely disappointed in her "selfish husband." Apparently, little Jane took away whatever emotional support they had to offer to one another, and both resented her arrival.

Mrs. Slowman maintained that she did not divorce her husband "for Jane's sake." Her husband used the same excuse. Meanwhile they competed for Jane's love; the mother showered Jane with passionate kisses, and her father did the same. When Mrs. Slowman gave birth five years later to a baby boy, he received little love and attention from his parents who were deeply involved with Jane. Jane's brother became a psychopathic youngster.

Meanwhile Jane received the brunt of her parents' ambivalent love. She became her mother's confessor and her father's lover. She had to lie to both of them, and felt guilty for her lies. She tried to "keep peace" at home, while she was getting more and more tense and more withdrawn. She worried about her parents and was afraid that they might kill one another, and she hated them for making her worry, and hated herself for hating them. She tried hard to please both of them; she was a model child afraid to hurt her parents' feelings, yet both of them were often angry with her, demanding more compliance and more love.

Jane grew sulky and tense, afraid to say what she thought and afraid to think what she thought. She developed compulsive rituals and a few phobias. She was afraid to go out, to speak loudly, to touch knives and so on. When I saw her, she was a mute catatonic.

Mother Versus Child

Mothers of schizophrenic children represent a variety of psychological types, but apparently they share the love-demanding attitude. Frustrated in childhood and disenchanted in their marriages, they perpetuate their childish love-demanding attitude and expect from their child (in most cases, the only child or their firstborn) all the love they have failed to receive elsewhere.

Mothers of schizophrenic children often neglect their own physical health and do it ostentatiously, widely publicizing their true or imaginary ailments. It seems rather immaterial to argue the point as to whether these mothers are truly sick or masochists or just pretending to be sick and suffering. For the child has no way of finding out whether his mother suffers from an acute heart ailment or is pretending. The child who becomes schizophrenic trusts his mother and takes her communications in good faith.

Schizogenic mothers are *overprotective* and restrict the child's freedom in a consistent way. Very little, if any, independent action is allowed schizophrenics in childhood, their steps are watched, planned, supervised, and restricted, and they are forced to become "model children."

The mother confuses the child by presenting herself as the tyrant who controls the entire family. She adopts a protective-hostile manner, telling the child that he is weak, sick, stupid, or ugly and that she must protect and care for him. Yet at the same time she presents herself as a self-sacrificing, suffering, almost dying person.

This tyrant-martyr ambivalence with constant accusation of ingratitude and incessant demands for appreciation is, as far as the content of communication goes, a "double bind" (Bateson et al., 1956). But the issues at stake are more than a matter of communication.

These mothers cannot tolerate any independence, any growth of the child, or any successes which they themselves do not bring about. They are possessive, controlling their child's life, and they demand from the child an unlimited amount of love, gratitude, and self-sacrifice for the self-sacrificing tyrant-martyr mother (see Davis, 1961; Foudraine, 1961; Lu, 1961, 1962; Weakland, 1960; Wolman, 1961, 1965b, 1966; Wynne and Rychoff, 1958; and many others).

The normal reaction to this kind of emotional extortion would be hate, but the preschizophrenic child is not able to express his hate toward those who are hurting him. For at the same time that the mother is destroying the child, she is constantly professing that she loves him. She makes him hate himself for feeling hostile toward his self-sacrificing protector. He becomes frightened and confused and forces himself to deny his true, hostile feelings. As Federn (1952) stated it, the frightened child is forced to *hypercathect his love objects at the expense of self-cathexis.*

The future schizophrenic starts his life like any other child, helpless and dependent on aid from the outside, yet he soon realizes that there is something wrong with his parents and he lives under a constant threat of losing his weak, dependent parents. And the harder the child tries to please them, the more they demand from him; the more he gives away his love to them, the sooner he exhausts his emotional resources and ends in a psychotic breakdown.

Mothers of schizophrenic children are *dictatorial, moralistic,* and *self-righteous.* They demand absolute obedience and conformity and when the preschizophrenic child behaves as any other child would, he is accused of being unfair, ungrateful, unjust, and cruel to his poor, sick, self-sacrificing mother.

Hill described the mothers of schizophrenics as follows: "These mothers were ill. They needed their sons and daughters to give them a reason for existence. These mothers are devastatingly, possessively all-loving of their child who is to be schizophrenic. The father was often aggressive, but this belligerence was that of a very unwilling agent of his wife" (1955, pp. 106-107).

Figure 1 compares normal and schizogenic families.

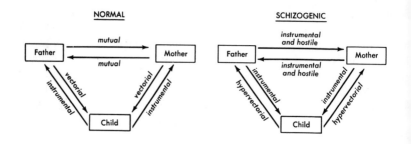

FIG. 1.   Normal and schizogenic families.

Clark (1961) studied the impact of interaction between mothers and their schizophrenic children on speech development. Some mothers avoided physical contact with their infants and communicated verbally before the child was ready for verbal communication. Consequently, the infant became withdrawn and unable to communicate either verbally or nonverbally, and remained mute and autistic. Some mothers, after giving birth to the child, become over-involved with him, renouncing all other pleasure-seeking outlets. These mothers indulged in intense physical contacts with the child and prevented him from relating to his peers and other people. The child spoke in a distorted, poorly articulate manner and became a symbiotic schizophrenic.

Esman et al. (1959) found that communication between parents and their schizophrenic child is seriously disturbed in many cases. These parents very often use their children for their own gratification of pregenital drives. The parents impair what is known as the separation-individuation phase of the child because they do not allow him to develop as an individual. The child turns to the alternative of autism or persistent symbiosis with the mother.

The typical parental attitudes toward the children who became schizophrenic have been described as follows (Wolman, 1966, pp. 79-83):

Mother *needs the child as a husband substitute.* By preventing the child's normal growth, mother prevents the child from leaving her. She conquers the child, takes it over, subjugates it to her own wishes and makes it into an obedient tool. Even when the child has grown up and married, mother doesn't loosen the bond.

The preschizophrenic child is not allowed to rebel. Were his mother outright hostile, it would be easier for him to rebel. Were she friendly, she would encourage his growth and independence. But mothers of schizophrenic patients are hostile in a friendly way. These mothers are colonial powers; they do not attack their children, but cut their wings; they make the child less of a person, undermine his self-confidence and demand more than the child is able to give. These mothers sharply criticize and tear the child down notwithstanding the effort he makes. Since they demand him to be what their husbands could not, their demands cannot be satisfied and the criticism goes on forever.

On a rainy day, one mother says, "*You* cannot go out because *you* will get sick right away." When the child brings good marks from school, the mother says, "Other children bring better marks." Overtly the mother is not hostile; she professes to be an idealistic and self-sacrificing mother. But she demands that the child be what she professes to be.

Whenever the child tries to act independently, mother resents it. Her love turns easily into hostility, into an accusing, blaming, devastating anger. Especially severe punishment was imposed when the child's loyalty shifted to the father; such a "betrayal" could not be accepted calmly by the mothers.

"A parent (normal or motherly) responds to a disturbance of a child by trying to relieve the disturbance. The narcissistic parent resents this disturbance and attacks the annoying aggressor (the child). The parental death-wish against the child may be perceived by the child's unconscious and constitute an 'unholy peril' with accompanying terrifying anxiety," wrote J. N. Rosen, a keen observer and daring therapist of schizophrenia. . . .

A truly vectorial mother can easily take the child's emotional difficulties. Since she genuinely loves the child, she tries to soothe his tension, allay anxiety, and calm anger. She would not punish a child because he was unhappy and cross. An instrumental mother attacks the child. No child can give his mother the affection and protection she needs. The disappointed mother becomes more demanding and hostile and the preschizophrenic child more and more disturbed.

Mother makes the child feel guilty because he cannot reciprocate for all the good things she does for him. Mother is a self-styled and self-advertising martyr and lures the child into a profound love and devotion. The bait she uses is her true or pretended self-sacrifice. "If I love you so much, the least you can do is try to make me happy," mother repeats. Since the child cannot possibly make mother happy, mother calls him selfish and ungrateful.

Here is the source of the so-called double-bind (cf. Bateson et al., 1956). Mother is instrumental and hostile, but pretends to be vectorial and friendly. The child often hates his mother and then hates himself for hating her. Mother complains that the child does not show initiative, does not play with other children, and does not separate from mother. But the preschizophrenic knows very well that mother would more resent his independence than she overtly resents his dependence. Mother needs him and cannot leave her. He is forced to become father's substitute; he is forced to take care of his poor mother or he will be exposed to her devastating accusations and his own guilt feelings.

The social roles related to age and sex are particularly important for mental health. Once we accept Freud's evolutionary developmental stages and theory of fixation and regression, the violation of the age-role becomes eo ipso a mental disorder. The emotional demands of mother force the child to abandon his social role of a little boy or a little girl. The preschizophrenic child begins to wonder: Is he male or female, a child or a parent? Who is he? Is he himself or his mother's agent? Is he a separate entity or part of his mother? Where are the boundaries? Is he allowed to have his own joys, sorrows, achievements, or must he sacrifice everything for his mother's sake?

It seems that the degree of mother's "colonialism" determines the severity of the disorder. Some mothers "bulldoze" the child into nothingness and create the autistic symptoms of early schizophrenia. Other mothers permit some degree of development, in which they parasitically control the child in the so-called symbiotic symptoms. Some are less forceful in their destructive protectiveness and schizophrenia develops gradually.

I do not know whether mother's attitude to the child suffices to drive him into schizophrenia, but the fathers of schizophrenics provide an additional and powerful push into the disorder.

Father versus child. Fathers are less complicated. They are frankly selfish, narcissistic, instrumental individuals. They have entered marriage with the desire and hope for being loved, admired and mothered. When they fail to obtain all that, they take on one of the four already mentioned positions of a sick, prodigious, rebellious, or runaway child. Obviously these fathers do not accept their social role of taking care of the children.

Many of these fathers resent being fathers and compete with their preschizophrenic children for the favors of their wives. One father was competing and fighting with his daughter at the dinner table for an additional serving of dessert. Another father was playing with his little son's toys. All these fathers tried to prove to their wives that they were nicer, better, smarter, or sicker than their children, and that they deserved all the attention the child was receiving.

One father used to display his drugs and medicines whenever his child was sick as if to say, "I am sicker than you." Another father did not approach the bed of his sick child out of fear of contagion. When a preschizophrenic child boasted his success in foreign language studies, his father started to study Latin to show his wife that he could master a more difficult language than his son did.

None of these fathers ever offered the child the usual paternal protection, control and discipline. Most of them ignored their children; some derided, teased, ridiculed, but none of them guided or helped. Most fathers did not care about their children, being always concerned with their own problems, hardships, or achievements.

Some fathers, especially of the more severe cases, were manifestly hostile to the child. Frustrated instrumentalism leads easily to overt hostility. When a preschizophrenic girl broke her leg and was brought home by neighbors, the irate father slapped her face for "what she was doing to him" (i.e., forcing him to take care of her). Some of the fathers were eager to beat the "bad child," either to please mother or to take revenge for the child's loyalty to mother, or without any apparent reason.

Some fathers acted seductively toward their own daughters. Since they failed in winning over their wives and could not force them to become "good mothers" to their own husbands, they turned to their daughters. It is always easier to play the role of the "hurt hero" with naive little girls than with adult women. One father physically attacked his wife because she molested "his" little girl. Many fathers indulged in sexual activities with their daughters and several of them hugged, kissed, and petted their teen-age daughters. Actual intercourse was more frequent in the lower socioeconomic class.

The fathers obviously wanted to be babied, were disappointed and therefore fought for the denied privileges. We already mentioned the four types of attitudes toward the wives. There has been even more variation in regard to children, inclusive of rejection, neglect, overt competition, hostility, and seductive efforts to win over the child and exploit it emotionally (sometimes also sexually) as a wife substitute.

Yet the patients disclosed little hatred toward their fathers. Father was perceived by the patients as a weak and friendly or weak and unfriendly individual, rejected or terrorized by mother. There has been a great deal of sympathy toward the "poor daddy," even when father was brutal.

The patients feared mother, feared her merciless demands and scolding criticism, but many of them tried very hard to elicit father's compassion. But even sickness could not bring the secondary gain of father's sympathy. The only way was to betray mother by becoming father's ally, companion, and eventually sex partner.

Thomes (1959) studied the problem of schizophrenics' parents with the use of:

1. The Parental Attitude Research Instrument (PARI), designed to measure a single attitude toward child rearing or family relationships.

2. Locke's Marital Adjustment Test, composed of questions on agreement and disagreement, satisfaction and common interests, of husband and wife.

3. Questions on certain aspects of parental role behavior, asking which parent was primarily involved in specific activities and decisions.

In this study, parents of 25 hospitalized schizophrenic children were compared with the parents of 25 normal children. Each case was matched by age and sex of the child, race, socioeconomic position of the family, and education of the parents.

The attitudes of mothers of schizophrenics as measured by the PARI did not differ from the attitudes of mothers of normal children; fathers of schizophrenics differed from the fathers of normal children on only 3 of the 23 scales.

Fathers of schizophrenics were more irritable and less inclined to communicate with their children than fathers of normals. Fathers of normal children were more inclined to protect their children from difficult experiences. These findings suggest that the fathers of schizophrenic children may provide a less satisfactory male figure with which the child may identify himself.

On marital adjustment, both mothers and fathers of schizophrenic children were less well adjusted than the mothers and fathers of normal children.

On role behavior, the mothers of schizophrenic children saw themselves more frequently as the person primarily responsible for certain activities with their child; while the mothers of normal children saw both themselves and their husbands as responsible for these activities.

According to Bettelheim (1967), the precipitating factor of infantile autism "is the parent's wish that his child should not exist" (p. 125). Accordingly, autism represents a defense on the part of the infant, erected to protect himself against an environment which he perceives to be totally annihilating. Because the parent does not want the child, he, the child, is not heard, and his cries become more and more impotent. Bettelheim believes the father "rarely is a main factor in childhood schizophrenia. His effect [the father's] is seen in all disturbances that begin after the third year of life. But in the early years, he is important only in regard to what he does or does not do for the mother and for the atmosphere he creates in the family home" (Bettelheim, 1967).

However, Eisenberg (1956) thinks that "the father has been the forgotten man. With little in the way of conclusive data to support the concept, the term 'schizogenic mother' has become almost a cliche of clinic usage, often perhaps not intended too seriously, yet nevertheless employed so freely as to indicate covert acceptance of this notion." Underlying this is the premise that the father is no less important a member of the family unit than his wife," both in terms of his direct influence on the child and of the fact that any inadequacy in the execution of his role is likely to affect the adequacy of the performance of the mother."

Apparently the etiology of schizophrenia "requires . . . the failure of the father to assume his masculine controlling function. . . . To produce schizophrenia it appears necessary for the mother to assume the father's role" (Whitaker, 1958, p. 108). "The parents follow a pattern very much like divorced parents who share their children. The mother, the overadequate one in relation to the inadequate child, is in charge of the child. . . . The father is then in the functioning position of a substitute mother" (Bowen, 1960, p. 363).

Often it is the father who triggers the tragic involvement with his child. He, too, expects the child to give him what he cannot get from his wife. He tends to become seductive toward children of both sexes, causing confusion with regard to age and sexual identification. Some fathers fight against their own wives and children, and many schizophrenic families live in fear of the angry father.

Manic depressives wish to be sick or dying in order to elicit their mother's love. They perceive their mother as a strong but hostile person whose sympathy and favors can be won only by weakness or illness. Schizophrenic children cannot expect anything in sickness; they are blamed for getting sick and burdening their mother.

Pathogenesis

Every parent of schizophrenic children himself wishes to remain a child. He or she married with the conscious or unconscious wish to be a child and to be taken care of by the marital partner. Sometimes these parents wish to have a child who could be their mate, friend, and confessor, but never a child who needs to be taken care of. A mother of a schizophrenic girl told her husband in my presence: "I wanted a child so you could take care of your *two little girls*. . . ."

If love means the desire to protect, to give, to care, no parent of a schizophrenic child has ever genuinely loved his child. All schizophrenic children are unwanted children born by a mishap, failure of contraceptives or a false desire to show that one is capable of having children. These children are viewed by their parents as burden and handicap, or as competitors in the desperate struggle to win a parental-type love of one's marital partner.

Since no man can become a father of his own wife and no woman can be her husband's mother, both parents are inevitably frustrated and hate one another. Marital life becomes a tug-of-war, in which the two parties hurt each other without being able to break away from one another. A man can divorce his wife, but a little boy cannot leave his beloved mommy. He can fight against mother and rebel against her, but ultimately he fights for her love. Failing in his efforts to win love, the husband hates his wife, and she hates him for failing her as a father substitute.

Everyone resents competitors. In schizogenic families the set of *social roles* has been reversed. The parents do not act like parents but like children; every one of them acts as if he were the other parent's child. The true child is viewed as an intruder who is often blamed for parental failures to act as adult marital partners and parents.

Hostile attitudes may lead to a variety of behavioral patterns. A straightforward death wish is merely one of the possible avenues. I came across several cases of schizophrenic children unfairly and severely punished by their parents. A self-righteous parent, disappointed in his (or her) marital partner, is prone to punish the child, using the child's minor transgression as an excuse for letting out pent-up hostility. I have seen schizophrenic children savagely beaten by their fathers and mothers; I have noticed more cruelty on the part of the fathers toward their sons and mothers toward their daughters.

Quite often schizogenic parents turn toward the child, expecting the child to compensate them for lack of marital love, in seductive heterosexual or homosexual advances. Sometimes these advances are partial and subtle, but sometimes they lead to genital or perverse sexual relations. It is more frequent between fathers and daughters than mothers and sons, and more often in lower than upper classes. Quite often these advances are directed by the parents toward the children of the same sex, thus adding confusion concerning sexual identity to the confusion about age and family position.

Overprotection is not love. Overprotecting mothers convey a message of distrust to the child. One mother stated succinctly: "My son Jimmy is such a nothing and a good-for-nothing, that I *must* take care of him." Another mother, who was washing and dressing her 12 year old schizophrenic daughter, complained: "Frances is unable to do anything by herself. Unless I wash her, she will stay dirty." The mother of a 19 year old schirophrenic used to wake him up in the morning, bring him his slacks and shirt, and comb his hair, maintaining that he was unable to perform the simplest chores. Very few schirophrenic girls are allowed to wash dishes or make beds, and those who do it are severely criticized for doing a poor job.

The child who becomes schizophrenic is exposed to demands he can never meet. He is supposed to do everything to please his parents, but nothing can really please them. Whenever he does whatever they want him to do, his efforts are taken for granted. Whenever he fails to please them, he is accused of being ungrateful and mean.

A normal child would rebel against such a treatment, but in a schizogenic family a true expression of resentment on the part of the child meets with never-ending accusations. The child is blamed for hurting his weak and self-sacrificing parents and is forced to feel sorry for those who rob him of his childhood. He is not allowed to remain a child, as instrumental as all other children. His immature parents force him to play the adult role of caring for them, and he becomes the parent of his parents. He is not allowed to enjoy childhood as other children do; he is not permitted to live his own life. His parents entangle him in their problems and emotional needs, and he becomes a *child without childhood*.

The severity of childhood schizophrenia depends on a variety of factors, and there is need for more detailed and more precise research. The available data of some authors quoted in this chapter, and some to be explained in further chapters, seems to indicate that *parental hostility and its timing* is of single greatest etiologic significance. When mother's verbal and nonverbal behavior conveys hostility to the infant in his first months of life, the infant's ego may never develop, and he may remain pseudo amentive or autistic. The milder the noxious factors and the later they appear, the milder the hypervectorial, schizo-type symptoms.

It seems that childhood schizophrenia starts in postnatal life in social interaction, affects personality development, and often causes physical disorders; it is therefore psychosomatic. The apparent physical symptoms and the tendency to develop various diseases could be interpreted as a psychosomatic expression of self-destructive tendencies. In a study of leukemic children, Baltrusch (1963) discovered that they were literally strangulated by maternal overprotection which was a cover-up for hidden hostility toward the child. Baltrusch hypothesized that leukemia may be viewed as "a physiologic response to certain patterns of withdrawal-conservation and that severe ego regressions may lead to ultimate somatic states of disorganization and exhaustion on a cellular level. Leukemia in this sense appears as a physiological pattern of decompensation in which the psychical state of decomposition has become expressed"

(Baltrusch, 1963, p. 180). These children, exposed to maternal hatred disguised as overprotection, wished to die.

Whether Baltrusch's hypothesis can be proven or not, the fact remains that schizophrenic children show a variety of physical symptoms, and these symptoms are probably the last link in the chain of the sociopsychosomatic deterioration process to be described in the following chapters.

CHAPTER 3

Schizophrenia in Early Childhood

1. INTRODUCTORY REMARKS

Some Earlier Studies

The study of childhood schizophrenia offers an invaluable opportunity for looking into the factors that lead to schizophrenia in adulthood. This study also broadens the scope of research into the peculiar dynamics of schizophrenic personality.

The problems of childhood schizophrenia have stirred up a great deal of controversy in regard to etiology, personality, dynamics, and even symptomatology. Some of these highly diversified points of view will be briefly reviewed here. (They were discussed in detail in Chapter 2.)

Sackler and associates (1952) related childhood schizophrenia to neuroendocrine factors. They found a high incidence of thyroid dysfunction in mothers, frequent endocrine dyscrasias, and suggested that an operative adrenocortical excess was related to the etiology and pathogenesis of schizophrenia. In all 19 cases studied by Sackler et al. the onset was before the age of four, and 13 children out of 19 were below the age of two.

Kanner (1943, 1946, 1949, 1955) introduced in 1943 the concept of "early infantile autism." Originally, Kanner believed in biological origins of autism, but when further research failed to support this point of view, Kanner turned to the study of parental attitudes. Lack of affection on the part of mothers and fathers was singled out by Kanner as the main causative factor. The overt behavior of autistic children has been described as dehumanized, mechanical, lacking vitality and spontaneity, and rigid and lifeless.

Research workers at the James Jackson Putnam Center called their little patients children with "atypical development" (Rank, 1949, 1955; Putnam, 1955; and others). The outstanding symptoms are "withdrawal from people, retreat into a world of fantasy, mutism or the use of language for autistic purposes, bizarre posturing, seemingly meaningless stereotyped gestures, impassivity or violent outbursts of anxiety and rage, identification with inanimate objects or animals, and excessively inhibited or excessively uninhibited expression of impulses" (Rank, 1955, pp. 491-492). The most important etiologic factors were related to "profound disturbance" in the early parents-child relationship and traumatic events, especially separation from parents (*ibid.*, p. 493).

This observation falls in line with what has been said in this matter by Bateson et al. (1956), Lidz et al. (1957, 1958, 1960), and others, and what was explained in detail in this volume in Chapter 2. Rank pointed to a "fragmented ego" that is "the result of the infant's unsuccessful struggle to obtain vital satisfaction from his parents" (Rank, 1955, p. 495). This "paralyzed ego" retreats into a world of fantasy and "co-exists" with the development of certain functions. This leads to the well-known disparity in development in schizophrenic children.

Overt Symptoms

Most research workers in this field believe that childhood schizophrenia is not exactly the same clinical entity as schizophrenia in adulthood. Bradley (1947) pointed to withdrawal from reality, escape into the world of fantasy, lack of social contacts, and improper emotional response as the outstanding symptoms of childhood schizophrenia. In addition, he noticed a decline in physical activity and exceeding sensitivity to criticism. Speech disturbances, fear of death, world destruction fantasies were observed by Despert (1955). Bender regards childhood schizophrenia as a "maturational lag at the embryonic level characterized by a primitive plasticity." Bender noticed vasovegetative, motor, emotional, social, perceptual, and intellectual disturbances (1942, 1947a, 1953, 1968).

The vasovegetative disorders include excessive flushing and perspiration, cold extremities, unpredictable reaction to physical illness, occasional high temperatures, disturbances in eating, sleeping, bowel and bladder control, disturbances in menstruation, etc. The motor abnormalities include oral and nasal mannerisms, awkwardness, fear of climbing stairs, of swinging, of riding a bicycle, and of any new motor activity. Some of these children display a tendency to whirl or rotate. The emotional disturbances include anxiety and apathy, and states of panic and bewilderment. Socially, these children are rather attractive, empathetic, and try to lean on or even incorporate the other person, be it a parent or therapist. Their perceptions are bizarre; primary and secondary processes are mixed together. They often use the third person pronoun instead of "I"; if there is speech, it is frequently disturbed. Schizophrenic children are preoccupied with problems of their own identity, of body and bodily functions. On the basis of her extensive studies, Bender has suggested dividing childhood schizophrenia into three types, namely, the autistic or pseudo-defective, the pseudo-neurotic, and the pseudo-psychopathic with paranoid ideas (Bender, 1956). And here is Bender's definition of the disorder of childhood schizophrenia:

"We now define childhood schizophrenia as a maturational lag at the embryonic level in all the areas which integrate biological and psychological behavior disturbance in all areas of personality functioning. It is determined before birth and hereditary factors appear to be important. It may be birth itself, especially a traumatic birth. Anxiety is the organismic response to this disturbance which tends to call forth symptom formation of a pseudo-defective, pseudo-neurotic, or pseudo-psychopathic type" (Bender, 1954, pp. 512-513).

There is no doubt that Bender's amassed empirical data are evidence of somatic disorders in childhood schizophrenia. However, lacking adequate proof of inherited and prenatal, intrauterine etiologic factors (cf. Chapter 2), one is inclined to view somatic symptoms as a *product* of psychological changes started by social causes. The occurrence of gastrointestinal and respiratory dysfunctions, allergies, and metabolic irregularities offers support to our socio-psychosomatic theory of schizophrenia. There is no evidence whatsoever that the infant's disturbed sleep, crying, screaming, and refusal to take food in the first months of life is inborn or inherited. Those research workers "who have taken part in well-baby clinics or in studies of personality development from birth on are keenly aware of the daily, almost hourly, shifts in a young infant's behavior, as manifested in tension or relaxation, in response to or coincident with tensions or relaxation in the mother. We have all seen newborn babies, who ate and slept quite peacefully in the hospital, go through periods of extreme upset at home" (Putnam, 1955, p. 521).

Valuable insights into the earliest childhood experiences have been offered by Despert (1951, 1952), Bettelheim (1950, 1955, 1967), Geleerd (1946, 1960), Mahler (1949, 1955, 1958, 1968), and many others that will be discussed later on.

Case Study Approach

Many years of observation of schizophrenic children in institutional settings (Institute of Disturbed Children, Poland; Institute for Therapeutic Education, Israel; and Jacobi Hospital, New York) and in private practice and studies of some of their families indicate that the type and symptomatology of childhood schizophrenia are largely determined by the pattern of the intrafamilial interaction or interindividual cathexis. Schizophrenia in infancy or *vectoriasis praecocissima* is a mental catastrophe that has taken place even before the ego has had the opportunity to grow and to assert control over the id.

The main difference between the infantile and adult schizophrenia lies apparently in *developmental factors*. Adult schizophrenics improve or deteriorate, while infant schizophrenics, in addition to having these ups and downs, are also subject to growth and maturation processes related to their age. These processes complicate the clinical picture.

All schizophreno-type symptoms are a downward adjustment for survival, but the morbid adjustment of a hurt child may go in more than one direction. As a result, there are several schizo-type behavioral patterns in childhood, depending on the age of the child, sex, severity of damage, level of development, specific family influences, etc.

An important distinction should be made at this point. Schizophrenia in adulthood is a failure of the impoverished ego that has lost most of its resources in object cathexis and has been hard-pressed ("overdemanded") by the superego to overcontrol its id. The failure of the ego to control the id indicates that the ego has ceased to be the steering wheel of the organism. In childhood hypervectorial disorders, the ego may have never had the chance to assume such a role. Childhood schizophrenia therefore cannot be viewed as a regressive process, but as a series of roadblocks erected on various points of the child's road to maturity.

The damage caused by a certain amount of stress corresponds to both the severity of stress and to the developmental stage of the child. However, it is not a case of simple arithmetic. Maternal hostility to a one year old normal infant may be devastating; it would definitely cause less harm if directed against an 11 year old normal child. However, if this 11 year old child has already had a great number of adverse conditions and is already highly disturbed, maternal hostility can be the straw that breaks the half-broken camel's back.

No human being acts all his life in exactly the same manner. Studies of family relations (Eisenberg, 1957; Jackson, 1960; Lidz et al., 1958; Wolman, 1961, 1965a; Wynne and Rychoff, 1958; and others) show that the same parent interacts in a different way with each child and is hardly, if ever, consistent in interaction with the same child. Statistical averages cannot do justice to the entire clinical truth, and there is no substitute for meticulous case studies that trace the particular listings of single cases. Generally speaking, the earlier the noxious experiences have taken place and, particularly, the most overt violence that has occurred in the family, the more severe is the child's disorder.

2. THE PSEUDO-AMENTIVE SYNDROME

Neonates

There is no evidence that the schizophrenic pattern must start at a definite developmental stage. It seems, however, that the earlier it starts, the more profound is the damage and the more difficult the therapy.

My longitudinal studies point in some cases to very early disbalances. Some cases of adolescent patients, where definite schizophrenic symptomatology was evident in early childhood, probably represent an "overstayed" childhood schizophrenia. There was then little if any regression, but there was much development from infancy to adolescence.

In some cases the praecocious hypervectorial (that is, schizophrenic) process starts at the oral stage. The infant apparently senses or empathizes his mother's demanding attitude and father's selfishness. Refusal to suck, vomiting, and sleep disturbances have been among the earliest symptoms that suggest the infant's fear of growing. Fear of eating, inability to chew food, avoidance of new foods, fear of biting, lack of assertiveness, lack of initiative have frequently been observed in infantile schizophrenia (Bettelheim, 1950; Ribble, 1938; and many others).

In these pseudo-amentive, very severe cases of infantile schizophrenia, development was stopped before it had the chance to start. It seems that all aspects of growth are affected, including motor coordination, homeostasis and metabolism, sleep and waking, food intake, speech, and mental development. Sometimes the process looks congenital, but in all the cases which I have studied in the last 30 years, the child was born normal, but the family pattern was schizogenic. Moreover, whenever the mothers of these children I observed received guidance or therapy, the child improved. "We all have seen newborn babies, who ate and slept quite peacefully in the hospital, go through periods of upset at home, and subsequently reassert their potential for easy normal behavior if and when it became possible for mother to modify her attitude favorable," wrote Putnam (1955, p. 521).

Pseudo-amentive schizophrenic children can be seen in mental hospitals attacking themselves, scratching their faces, and tearing their hair. Some of them, apparently fixated at the oral-aggressive stage, swallow their hair. One little girl developed severe digestive trouble when the swallowed hair formed a huge lump in her stomach. Hospital aids had to tie the hands of a four year old boy or to watch him constantly after he severely scratched his face and almost pulled out his own eyes.

Pseudo-amentives suffer a variety of physical diseases. Many of them cannot swallow solid food and have to be bottle-fed. Some of them throw up any food, choke even on fluids, and cannot digest their food. Their metabolic condition is severely disturbed, and they often fall prey to respiratory diseases.

One of the main symptoms of these pseudo-amentive infants is severe mental deficiency, and many of these pseudo-idiotic children are frequently institutionalized as mentally defectives. Richards (1951) found 22 cases of schizophrenic children in an institution for mental defectives. One of my first patients was diagnosed as a severe imbecile and was put among mentally retarded children. This pseudo-amentive schizophrenic partially responded to psychological treatment and his responses to mental tests showed an amazing improvement after one year.

Gesell and Amatruda stressed institutional impact on "pseudo symptomatic retardation." "It is symptomatic because it is the immediate expression of causative factors operating at the time of diagnosis" (Gesell and Amatruda, 1947, p. 136). The authors describe the excessive amount of discontinuity in institutions "particularly with respect to personal contacts and relationships. The result is a feebled sense of security and blurred sense of identity" (*ibid.*, p. 322). Table 1 represents the order of appearance of adverse reactions in institutional infants as listed by these authors.

Goldfarb (1961) tested institutionalized schizophrenic children with a battery of tests, and his results are shown in Table 2.

TABLE 1
Institutionalization

	Approximate Age of Appearance
1. Diminished interest and reactivity........................	8-12 weeks
2. Reduced integration of oral behavior.....................	8-12 weeks
3. Beginning retardation evidenced by disparity between exploitation in supine and in sitting situations................	12-16 weeks
4. Excessive preoccupation with strange persons..............	12-16 weeks
5. General retardation (prone behavior realtively unaffected)....	24-28 weeks
6. Blandness of facial expression...........................	24-28 weeks
7. Impoverished initiative.................................	24-28 weeks
8. Channelization and stereotypies of sensori-motor behavior....	24-28 weeks
9. Ineptness in new social situations........................	44-48 weeks
10. Exaggerated resistance to new situations..................	48-52 weeks
11. Relative retardation in language behavior.................	12-15 months
12. Definite improvement with improvement of environment	

TABLE 2

Neurological Test Scores for Normal and Schizophrenic Children*

	Normal		Schizophrenic		Difference Between Means
	Mean	s	Mean	s	Means
Double simultaneous stimulation with eyes closed (number correct)†	4.0	—	3.1	1.2	0.9
With eyes closed, heterologous (number correct)†	9.6	1.1	5.2	4.6	4.4
With eyes open, homologous (number correct)	3.9	0.5	3.2	0.9	0.7
With eyes open, heterologous (number correct).x	7.2	2.8	3.8	4.5	3.8
Total score	25.1	3.9	15.3	10.5	9.8
Oculomotor functioning (rating)	8.4	0.9	5.7	2.1	2.7
Muscle tone (rating)	2.7	0.5	2.1	0.6	0.6
Whirling, arms at sides (rating)	18.0	1.9	13.8	4.8	4.1
Whirling, arms outstretched and parallel (rating)	13.1	1.5	8.5	2.6	4.6
Romberg, arms at sides (rating)	26.4	2.2	16.7	8.0	9.7
Romberg, arms outstretched and parallel (rating)	12.6	3.7	10.6	3.7	2.0
Finger-to-finger (rating)	3.8	0.5	2.6	1.6	1.2
Finger-to nose (rating)	3.9	0.3	2.4	1.6	1.5

*By means, standard deviations, differences between normals and schizophrenics, and significance of difference between means of groups.

†The maximum score for homologous stimuli is 4, and for heterologous stimuli is 10.

Some children Goldfarb called "untestable"; he had to exclude them from the test of the following reasons:

1. Genuine incapacity for the task.

2. Reasons other than incapacity: (a) Poor comprehension. The child's behavior suggested that he was trying but could not understand what he was expected to do despite repeated demonstration and every effort to simplify directions for him. (b) Inattention. The child was not able to attend to the task because of his distractability

by inner and outer stimuli. (c) Inability to sustain effort. The child was unable to persist at a given task for the time required. (d) Resistance. The child was uncooperative and consciously or unconsciously, resisted complying with directions.

Goldfarb concluded:

> Schizophrenic children and normal children matched for age and sex did not differ in basic physical characteristics such as height, weight, and sensory acuity. Normals were superior to schizophrenics in neurological functioning, as appraised by patterned neurological functions; in qualitative aspects of behavior such as activity, attention, and sustained effort; in perception; in conceptualization; in psychomotor response; and in speech and communication. Schizophrenic children were more likely to be uncertain about their self-identity, with attendant confusion in time, space, person, and body schema. They also showed aberrant receptor behavior characterized by extremes of hyper- or hyposensitivity and by receptors of hearing and vision.

Schizophrenic children excluded from Goldfarb's neurological study were called "organic." The issue of organicity has often been revised in recent research literature for many schizophrenic children, especially in regard to the very severe cases called by me pseudo-amentive, who display a galaxy of physical symptoms.

The diversity of physical symptoms militates, however, against a single organic etiology. Etiologic issues were scrutinized in Chapter 2, but it is worth mentioning here that organic symptoms could be psychosomatic, and that their genetic origin has never been proved.

On the other hand, there is a growing body of evidence related to the impact of severe emotional deprivation on the child's physical and mental growth. Goldfarb himself, in a study of emotional deprivation in the first year of life, proved that deprivation of mothering may cause damage beyond repair to the child's development; this damage cannot be interpreted by hereditary factors (Goldfarb, 1945a, 1945b).

Failure in Mothering

The nature of symptoms depends primarily on the nature of offense. Some children have been exposed to a schizogenic family interaction from the day they were born or the day they came home from the maternity hospital. From that day on, they sensed or empathized or somehow were made to feel that mother did not want them because *she herself wanted to be taken care of*. One mother of a schizophrenic five year old child reported that when her husband visited her in the maternity ward, she said: "Now you have to take care of two children. Don't forget me. I am your first child. You must love both of us."

This woman felt resentful toward the infant when he disturbed her husband's sleep. The neonate, so she said, was breaking up the family, disturbing marital relations, and demanding too much attention. The woman wondered why her girl friend's infant slept quietly while her own child was restless. From the very first days she had feeding difficulties. She did not realize that her unconscious competition with the infant and her hostile attitude caused severe anxiety and gastrointestinal and homeostatic troubles in the infant. She complained as follows:

As far back as I can recall, the child was peculiar, sensitive, touchy, cranky, crying, restless, and demanding all the attention. I had to sacrifice everything for him. He did not let me go out. He refused to eat and vomited frequently. Quite often he did not go to sleep and screamed for hours. I had to spend days and nights with the baby. I neglected my husband and we began to quarrel. This child has brought discord and unhappiness to our home. We had our difficulties and occasional squabbles before he was born, but since that time life has become torture. I decided to sacrifice my life for my child, and suffered in a stoic manner. But then I realized how selfish my husband was. I became mother and father to my poor child. I knew that I had to take care of everything, all alone, neglected by my selfish husband, isolated from everybody, alone in my tragedy. Soon, I began to resent the child. I wished he were not born, yet I had to take care of him, take care of the little idiot.

Needless to say, the mother *reversed the causal order;* her unwillingness to take care of her child, related to her wish to be taken care of herself, caused the child's troubles, which in turn made her resent him more and more.

The schizophrenic child is not the "rejected" child, for a schizogenic mother does care. But she takes care in an extremely hostile and pseudo-vectorial manner. Her motherly care is an exercise in yelling, crying, screaming, beating, and forcing food down the child's throat "for his well-being." Often she will go on in a tirade to the infant in the crib: "Why can't you sleep? See how tired I am. You are the worst child ever born!"

I saw this child in my office. He did not talk, did not feed himself, refused solid food, and was not toilet-trained at the age of five. He frequently whined, whimpered, rocked, banged his head, scratched his face, and pulled and swallowed his hair.

Apparently human infants need a friendly attitude, love and affection no less than they need milk. Those who love cathect their libido in their love objects; those who are loved receive these cathexes. Human infants cannot love without love.

Ribble (1938) has described cases of total rejection of newborn infants by their mothers. In some cases, the infants fell into a stupor and had to be treated as if in a coma. Spitz (1945) studied 61 infants in a foundling home where one nurse took care of too many infants. The hygiene, physical care, and the precautions against contagious diseases were impeccable, yet the infants showed an unusual susceptibility to infection. Of a total of 88 infants below the age of $2\frac{1}{2}$, 23 died. In one ward (age 18 to 30 months), only two out of 26 surviving infants could say a few words; out of the same 26, two could walk. All the infants performed poorly on Hetzer-Wolf infant developmental tests. Spitz explained that inadequate perceptual development was caused by lack of emotional supplies. In our terms, it was the lack of interindividual object cathexis from parent to child. In Spitz's words, "Our thesis is that perception is a function of libidinal cathexis and, therefore, the result of the intervention of an emotion of one kind or another. Emotions are provided for the child through the intervention of a human partner, i.e., by the mother or her substitute." (Spitz, 1945, pp. 67-68). I believe that it was not only the lack of perceptive stimuli that caused the arrest in normal physical and mental growth, but the lack of parental love. The infant, as it were, was *frightened away from normal growth*.

Adult schizophrenics, afraid to face normal life, regress into infantile behavior. Schizophrenia in adults is a morbid downward adjustment for survival. Infantile schizophrenics are paralyzed by fear to live, and they *refuse to grow up*. Their apparent inhibition of emotional and intellectual growth is a sort of downward adjustment. They seem to build a shell and try to hide in the shell, avoiding threatening contacts.

All other factors being equal, the earlier the damage is caused, the more severe it is. As mentioned before, the severity of the initial offense, and of subsequent ones, is an important factor in the course of disorder and its severity. Most of the ambulatory or hospitalized adult schizophrenics have had some years of close to normal or neurotic life, but infantile schizophrenics have never been normal or even neurotic. Their ego was squashed before it had the chance to develop. There were no chances for developing ego protective, that is, neurotic, symptoms. Infantile psychosis or *vectoriasis praecosissima* usually starts in the first year of the infant's life. Sometimes it is so severe that it affects practically everything: emotions, motility, over-all personality structure, intellectual functions, metabolism, physical growth, etc. It is a downward adjustment from human life to a vegetative life; it is, as all types of schizophrenia are, an effort to survive on a lower evolutionary level.

Total Emotional Deprivation

A complete lack of mothering has been often linked to the most severe syndrome of infantile schizophrenia. Institutional rearing of infants, called by Spitz "hospitalism," has been defined as "vitiated conditions of the body due to long confinement in a hospital, or the morbid condition of the atmosphere of a hospital" (Spitz, 1945, p. 53).

In the above-mentioned study Spitz investigated the following aspects of development (Spitz, 1946b, p. 113):

1. Bodily performance: the gross indicator used was whether the child could sit, stand, or walk.

2. Intellectual capacity to handle materials: the gross indicator was whether the child was capable of eating food alone with the help of a spoon, and whether he could dress alone.

3. Social relations: these were explored by ascertaining the number of words spoken by each child, and by finding out whether he was toilet trained."

And here follow the results of his investigations:

1. Bodily development:
   Incapable of any
      locomotion   5
   Sit up unassisted
      (without walking)   3
   Walk assisted   8
   Walk unassisted   5
                   Total   21

2. Handling materials:
   Cannot eat alone with
      spoon   12
   Eat alone with spoon   9
                   Total   21

3. Adaptation to demands of
   environment:
   Not toilet trained in
      any way   6
   Toilet trained,
      partially   15
                   Total   21

4. Speech development:
   Cannot talk at all   6
   Vocabulary: 2 words   5
   Vocabulary: 3 to 5
      words   8
   Vocabulary: a dozen
      words   1
   Uses sentences   1
                   Total   21

Spitz says (*ibid.*, pp. 114-115):

As seen from these data, the mental development of these 21 children is extraordinarily retarded, compared to that of normal children between the ages of two and four, who move, climb, and babble all day long, and who conform to or struggle against the educational demands of the environment. This retardation, which amounts to a deterioration, is borne out by the weights and heights of these children, as well as by their pictures.

Normal children by the end of the second year weigh, on the average, 26½ pounds, and the length is 33½ inches. At the time of this writing, 12 of the children in Foundling Home range in age between 2.4 and 2.8; 4, between 2.8 and 3.2; and 5, between 3.2 and 4.1. But of all of these children, only 3 fall into the weight range of a normal two-year-old child, and only 2 have attained the length of a normal child of that age. All others fall below the normal two-year level—in one case, as much as 45 per cent in weight and 5 inches in length. In other words, the physical picture of these children impresses the casual observer as that of children half their age.

During the second half of the first year, 15 per cent of the infants began to develop an unusual sequence of behavior. They cried continuously, but after several months the crying subsided and they became indifferent to adults. "The children would lie or sit with wide-open, expressionless eyes, frozen immobile face, and a faraway expression as if in a daze, apparently not perceiving what went on in their environment" (Spitz, 1946a, p. 314).

This behavior was called by Spitz "anaclitic depression," for it resembled severe adult depression. In many cases, this unusual behavior began to develop after the child was separated from its mother or mother substitute. If favorable mother-child relationships were reestablished within three months, a more normal course of development occurred.

Infants at the age of six to eight months separated from their mother for two months refuse contact, lie supine in their cribs with very little motion, sometimes wail, lose weight, retard in motor coordination; their facial expression becomes rigid. They are prone to contract a variety of diseases with little chance to survive them. At the age of four these children could not sit, stand, walk, and talk. Their I.Q. was below 45. At the age of two 35 per cent of these infants died and this mortality rate continued unabated.

Bakwin thus summarized the effect of deprivation in motherly care (1949, p. 513):

> Infants under six months of age who have been in an institution for some time present a well defined picture. The outstanding features are listlessness, emaciation and pallor, relative immobility, quietness, unresponsiveness to stimuli (like a smile or coo), indifferent appetite, failure to gain weight properly despite the ingestion of diets which in the home are entirely adequate, frequent stools, poor sleep, an appearance of unhappiness, proneness to febrile episodes and absence of sucking habits.

Theoretical Explanations

The theoretical explanation of the *pseudo-amentive schizophrenic* follows the principles explained in Chapter 1 of this volume. All human children are born helpless and in dire need of help. They wake up when hungry, thirsty, cold, wet, or in pain. When their needs are satisfied by a loving mother, they fall asleep in a happy mood called "bliss" by Freud and "euphoria" by Sullivan. Apparently infants empathize and somehow perceive the affectionate vectorial parental attitude; they get tense and anxious when they get milk without love.

Schizogenic parents or parental substitutes are not vectorial. They provide care and give food, but they are unable to give love. An extreme and early lack of love on the part of the parents or parental substitutes plays havoc with the infant's somatopsychic structure. Schizophrenia in adults is caused by a lavish libido cathexis in one's love objects with resulting impoverishment of the ego. The preschizophrenic child gives away too early and too much love to his parents, and therefore not enough libido is left for self (ego) cathexis. The impoverished ego develops a galaxy of symptoms and, ultimately, heads toward a psychotic collapse.

The earliest childhood schizophrenia, called pseudo-amentive vectoriasis praecocissima, starts *before* the ego has been formed. The infant receives no or very little libido cathexes from without. A distinct unwillingness to take care of him or a veiled wish to get rid of him is communicated to him in a nonverbal way. The infant senses, empathizes, or somehow perceives that he is unwanted, and that his mother and often father wish him dead.

The only possible way to survive is to stop growth and, if possible, to withdraw to *prenatal life*. Prenatal life was the only protected and safe period of life, and regression to this stage seems to be the only way for survival. An adult schizophrenic's behavior is guided by an unspoken motto: "If I canot live as a normal adult, I shall try to survive by regressing to infantile modes of behavior." The pseudo-amentive schizophrenic child regresses into prenatal life.

The most severe cases of severe childhood schizophrenia seen by Spitz, Putnam, Bender, myself, and others resemble fetal life in its avoidance of activities. The intrauterine motor activity is limited and the general forms of life are rather restricted. Pseudo-amentive infants rock and bang their hands, but this is rather limited activity in scope and initiative. They are not suicidal in this behavior; they seem to conserve their energy and, as it were, refuse to grow in the open world.

Maternal hostile instrumentalism forces the infant to give up growth and development. Pseudo-amentive symptoms start as early as the first few weeks of life. Bergman and Escalona (1949) described early sensitivity in infants and hypothesized innate factors. There is no reason to hypothesize genetic factors when there is an apparent maternal unwillingness to take care of the neonate. Mental life starts before birth, and in prenatal life mother's organism acts in a vectorial manner giving the fetus all the required supplies. Irrespective of mother's moods and wishes, the intrauterine life offers maximum security. To be born is always a traumatic experience, and it takes a great deal of tender love and maternal care to help the infant to adjust to extrauterine life.

The pseudo-amentive child is the child who has failed to obtain this help. The message he got is clear and cruel: "No one wants you."

3. AUTISTIC SCHIZOPHRENIA

The second stage of infantile schizophrenia is autism. The terms autism, autistic, etc., have been used loosely in description of a variety of withdrawal symptoms, peculiar behavior, and inadequate mental development. In the present book the term autism is used as a name of a cluster of symptoms that accompany a severe schizophrenia in infancy, second in gravity to the pseudo-amentive syndrome.

Autistic thinking was first studied in 1913 by E. Bleuler. Bleuler defined autistic thinking as "turning away from reality, and seeing life in fantastic pictures" (Bleuler, 1913, p. 874). Autistic individuals live in their dream world, imagining that their needs have been gratified, while they are not.

Once a father and a mother came to my office with a $3\frac{1}{2}$ year old boy. The mother was an ambitious young lady who had graduated from a school of higher learning and was holding an important scientific position. She was married to an unambitious, indecisive, meek man. She was bitterly disappointed in marriage and highly critical of her husband. The husband complained that his wife was domineering, unfair to him, and unfriendly. Her constant criticism had undermined his self-confidence, causing him to fail in business. The child did not talk and could not eat by himself, but he was perfectly toilet trained. The mother said that she had "sacrificed" years of her scientific career taking care of "the big idiot" (husband) and now "this little idiot, too." Sixteen months earlier she had decided that she had "had enough" of sitting home and had taken up her career. She believed herself to be highly conscientious, a warm, affectionate, and giving person, caught in marriage to a stupid man, and a mother to an infant monster. Her burning desire was to get rid of both and be free again. She felt guilty, however, about her death wish in regard to both. She had decided to remain married "for the sake of the child," whom she hated and overprotected, resented and manipulated.

She did not hide her feelings. Her confessions, made in my office in the presence of both husband and child, were full of accusations and curses thrown in the face of her husband. She did not hide her feeling for the child, crying loudly, "This child kills me; he is a killer."

A pseudo-amentive child is a child whose maturation process has been prevented in the first months of life by parental hostile instrumentalism. Early autism is not a complete refusal to grow; it is withdrawal and regression. An autistic child is a child whose ego was badly damaged before it had the opportunity to protect the system. *Pseudo-amentive schizophrenia is a regression to prenatal life; autism is a regression of the infantile ego into the id.* An autistic child is a child whose libido has been stolen from him in object hypercathexis and has been forced to turn inward, yet some initial development has already taken place and the child's overt behaviour is one step ahead of pseudo-amentive schizophrenic.

Here is a brief description of another autistic child, mute, withdrawn and self-mutililating. The mother was a disciplinarian and severely punished the one year old infant for soiling. She forced him to refrain from crying and expressing protest and hostility. She beat him for soiling; she punished him for crying; whenever he cried, she hit him; she hit him again for screaming with pain and left him alone when he was whimpering. She came back after a few minutes with a vehement and malicious tirade against the "bad boy who is as wicked as his hoodlum father." Yet even in rage she never neglected the physical needs of the infant. He was fed, changed, washed, and received all the necessary hygenic care, accompanied by blows and words of hate. The infant never learned to speak. His eyes and his face had an intelligent expression, but he did not talk. He probably understood a lot of things, but never dared to speak.

Freud related autistic thinking to the unconscious, while Bleuler believed that autistic thinking can be either conscious or unconscious.

Kanner introduced the concept of infantile autism. In 1944, Kanner described 11 cases of infantile autism. Five of them were firstborn, three only children, one the oldest of three, one the younger of two, and one the youngest of three siblings.

Initially Kanner distinguished between autism and schizophrenia, but later (1949) he found that childhood schizophrenia may develop from infantile autism. The common denominator of all cases of infantile autism was the infant's inability to relate to people, their "acting as if people weren't there," their autistic aloneness that 'shuts out anything that comes to the child from the outside' " (Kanner, 1960, p. 717). Nearly two-thirds of these children learned to speak, but language, wrote Kanner, did not serve for communication with others; therefore, "there is no essential difference between the speaking and the mute children." There was an absence of spontaneous sentence formation and echolalia type of reproduction. Kanner pointed to their apathy, withdrawal from social contacts, obsessive insistence on routine and sameness, fear of change, lack of speech or disordered speech, and talking about themselves in the third person. Occasionally, these children displayed spectacular memory.

In a follow-up study of 42 autistic children, Kanner and Eisenberg (1955) found that at the average age of 14 most of them retained the early characteristics but lost some symptoms such as echolalia and pronominal reversals. Of the nonspeaking children, 18 out of 19 remained in a state of complete isolation and were hardly distinguishable from mentally defective children. Children who have not learned to talk by four years of age are prognostically bad cases. Eighteen out of the 19 nonspeaking children showed no improvement whatsover.

The 23 children who used language represented in the follow-up a more encouraging picture. No less than 13 out of 23 have been able to function at home and in the community, although they were still schizoids and maintained a tenuous contact with reality. Especially illuminating is the case of George, a mute four year old autistic boy. In his case, therapeutic emphasis was put on the mother. The mother responded very well and "took George over as a challenge . . . after a year, George began to use language . . . now, approaching his twelfth birthday, he is about to be promoted to the sixth grade" (*ibid.,* p. 235).

Normal children make anticipatory motor adjustments when picked up, whereas autistic children do not show any interest. The autistic child, when picked up or moved to another position, responds slowly or not at all. Autistic children display excellent rote memory; thus in some cases I saw the parents show off with the child's spectacular recitations of things parents gave them to memorize. Autistic children memorize words they do not understand and cannot utilize. When spoken to, an autistic child tends to repeat what has been said to him (echolalia) and he uses personal pronouns the way he hears them. As a result, he may talk about himself in the second or third person.

In an autistic child the desire for sameness is an obsession. Autistic children fear change in their environment. They may play with things for hours happily, but become very angry when they do not fit in a given space. When left alone they are unaware of people in the same room. Should an adult disturb them with a question or touch an object of theirs, they fly into rage. An autistic child moves around in a group like a total stranger with recognition of no one. He is still oblivious of other children and plays by himself. Autistic children possess a better relationship to pictures of people than to people themselves. The expressions on their faces show extreme serious-mindedness or a sense of tenseness, but when alone with objects they like they tend toward a soft placid smile.

The main characteristic of an autistic child appears to be extreme aloneness from the very beginning of life, and therefore they do not respond to anything that comes to them from the adult world. They appear to be intelligent enough, providing nothing jeopardizes their opposition to change. Adult schizophrenics gradually withdraw, but autistic children are children and they are driven by *two opposite processes of morbid alienation of schizophrenia and normal development of socialization,* As they grow older, some of them venture into the open world, their language becomes more communicative, and they may even learn to use personal pronouns properly. Some of them try to cooperate with their environment and obey commands put forth to them. Normal children learn to eat new foods, walk by themselves, sing a new song, and play with new toys. Autistic children resist change and learn slowly and reluctantly.

Developmental Sequences

In a recent study of infantile autism (Ornitz and Ritvo, 1968) the following symptoms have been distinguished. In the first few months of life the autistic infant is either inactive or irritable or alternates between the two extremes. In this period there is no eye contact, no crying or smiling. In the second six months there is a "proprioceptive and antigravity" response against being tossed in the air. The infant shows no interest in toys, is afraid of rough-textured food, and any change in light and loud sounds may lead to a panic state. Motor development is either too slow or too fast; sometimes there is a distinct motor regression.

In the second year of life the autistic child shows an unusual sensitivity to auditory, visual, tactile, and "labyrinthine" stimulation. Rubbing and scratching surfaces seems to be his reaction to tactile stimuli. Repetitive habits develop in the second and third year. There may be a hyperextension of the neck, whirling, looking at objects, walking on toes, and staring.

DeMyer et al. (1967) compared 30 autistic and 30 normal children ranging in age from two to seven years as reported by their mothers in a questionnaire. Sex, race, religion, order of birth, and socioeconomic factors were controlled, and there were nine categories describing the aspects of play activity. Mothers of autistic children reported less complex toy play and a greater degree of perservative and nonconstructive play. Mothers' reports were corroborated by laboratory observations. Autistic children had elementary graphic skills like normal peers but did not draw recognizable figures, and there was less block play at all age levels. Autistic children's plays were less imaginary, and there was a great deal of throwing things and pounding.

Hutt and Ounsted (1966) studied the gaze fixation in eight autistic children aged three to six years and six nonautistics. Using pictures of happy, sad, blank, monkey, and dog faces, Hutt and Ounsted found that autistic children gazed at blank and animal faces most frequently. Most of the children stared at the light switches and windows. The happy face was chosen least frequently since it was probably associated with social demands. Autistic children did not explore faces and avoided them by peripheral vision and fractional glances.

A vivid description of autistic behavioral patterns was given by Norman (1955). While these children apparently failed to respond to human affection, their avoidance of human contact was neither complete nor absolute. These children are unable to look straight in someone's eyes and are tense when stared at but they may accept close physical contact in being held, hugged, and cared for by a friendly adult. The close physical contact seems to increase the child's feeling of identity.

Tilton and Ottinger (1964) compared the use of toys by autistic, mentally retarded, and normal children. Observations were made during 20 minute play periods where the children were allowed to select and use toys. The mean age for the autistic, retarded, and normal children was five years, five years and one month, and four years and ten months respectively. Normal children excelled the retarded in the use of toys. All normal children, 10 of the 12 retarded children and five of the 13 autistic children combined the toys in their play. Most autistic children used the toys in an oral and repetitive manner. They shook, knocked, twirled, and spun the toys, and their behavior was more "stereotyped than functional."

Mutism and Speech Disturbances

I have followed the life stories of several autistic children in institutions overseas and in this country. I have come to relate mutism and speech disorders to mother-child interaction. The life story of little Dorothy is a case in point. I had the chance to see the child and the parents frequently for a period of years.

The mother was in her middle thirties, the father about seven years older. They hated each other intensely. The mother continuously complained that her husband was a failure, insulted him frequently in my presence, ordered him around, and refused to sleep with him because "he didn't deserve her." The father was a bright man. As an electrical engineer he was quite successful, but unable to relate to people and meek and, therefore, judging by his abilities, rather an underachiever. He maintained that his wife's criticism had destroyed his self-confidence.

Dorothy was born against her father's will. The mother maintained that she wanted a child "to prove" that she was a woman. The birth of the child was, however, felt as a burden. The mother could not stay in bed until noon as she was used to, or watch late late shows on TV. She was impatient in feeding the child and angry when Dorothy did not finish the bottle of milk.

The father hired nurses, and the mother quarreled with and fired them. Soon the father became mother's unwilling assistant. Early morning and after work he fed the infant and changed diapers. On weekends the mother demanded rest from "the little monster," and the father took the baby out.

The infant did not speak at all. When I saw Dorothy she was two years old, retarded in motor development, mute, pale looking, and overweight. Pretty soon it became clear that mother *rarely if ever spoke to the child,* except for occasional shouting and cursing. She avoided the child as much as was physically possible. When she spoke to her husband about the child, she rarely called Dorothy by her name; it was always "she," the "nasty, stubborn, monstrous kid," that the mother complained about.

Dorothy cried often but it was rather whimpering and whining than crying. The mother could not stand that "whining monster" and yelled, "Shut up!" Dorothy did shut up, sitting for hours in a corner, staring, or banging toys her father bought her.

I started speech lessons with Dorothy by showing pictures and naming them. I repeatedly said, "You are nice, Doddy." I insisted that the parents talk to her; the mother never did it, but the father followed my instruction religiously, and by the age of four Dorothy spoke, but her articulation was poor and pronunciation faulty.

Mutism in autistic children was interpreted by L. Jackson (1950) as an effort to be immobile and to feign death. Feigning death is one of the primitive mechanisms of escaping a terrifying threat. Some adult catatonics in remission or recovery explained their mutism as a protective device: "If I keep my mouth shut, I cannot say anything wrong, and they will not blame me" (Wolman, 1966).

Speech and Language

Cunningham (1966) studied the language of an autistic boy. In the first six months of observation and at 24 months and at 30 months, the mean lengths of the sentences were 1.9 and 3.0 respectively. There was an advance in the first year in the variety of words, and then no improvement beyond the 30 month level. Articulation was at times poor and at times clear. Cunningham compared the performance of his little subject to McCarthy's (1930) study of normal language samples of 18 month to $4\frac{1}{2}$ year old children. In the speech of the autistic child: (1) articles were frequently missing, (2) certain verbs were often omitted, (3) pronouns and prepositions were often left out, and (4) there were very few questions. The examiner's questions were often ignored or repeated in monotone.

Apparently there is no one speech pattern for all schizophrenic children. Goldfarb and Mintz (1961) used observations of speech as a way of studying ego functions. They wrote: "Schizophrenic children have not achieved culturally expected patterns in such aspects of phonation, rhythm, articulation, gestural communication, and communication of mood and meaning. These defects, especially those in connotative communications, secondarily seemed to increase the social isolation of these children" (*ibid.*, 1961, p. 113). Schizophrenic children use neologisms, mix words up, and disarrange them, which makes it difficult for the listener to understand them (Eisenson, 1938).

Studies of adult schizophrenics show similar speech patterns. The adult schizophrenics, especially hebephrenics, mix words up in the same way as well as confusing parts of speech (Burstein, 1961; Wolman, 1966). The severity of psychosis can be determined to some extent by the various speech levels (Gottschalk, 1961).

In Kanner's study (1946), eight of 23 autistic children were mute, but these mute children occasionally spoke whole sentences. They spoke in a manner seemingly irrelevant to the situation, evidently making analogies and using metaphors. The metaphors used were "rooted in concrete, specific, personal experiences of the child who uses them" (Kanner, 1946, p. 243). This "metamorphical substitution" is common in autistic children.

According to Kanner, autistic speech may appear irrelevant and nonsenical but is actually a metamorphical expression which stands for various figures of speech where one thing is meant to stand for another which it resembles. There are several ways in which this transfer can occur. Thus, for instance, "Bread basket becomes 'home bakery'; Annette and Cecil become 'red' and 'blue,' and a penny becomes 'that's where we play ten pins.' " Sometimes the substitution is accomplished by generalization: " 'Home bakery' becomes the term for *every* basket; 'Don't throw the dog off the balcony' assumes the meaning of self-admonition in every instance when the child feels the need for admonishing himself."

Language serves communication, but autistic children do not necessarily want to be understood by others. The reversal of pronouns, one of the most definite symptoms of infantile autism, bears witness to the peculiarities of their language. All the autistic children I have ever seen confused pronouns in a way similar to catatonic echolalia. Little Dorothy for a long time talked about herself as "she," her mother as "I," and her father as "you."

A tape recorder was used by Pronovost (1961) in a study of speech of autistic children. One child in his study used sounds rather than words. When shown pictures of animals, the child tried to name them but was unable to do so because of his articulation limits. He was unable to articulate; probably the motor apparatus was not developed adequately. This child could match, after learning, the written word with the proper picture. Communicative speech was used to imitate the therapist in an echolalic sense.

Pronovost tried to test the language comprehension of autistic children. He devised a special scale, and found that autistic children understood more than was expected and recognized people's names, objects, and actions. Pronovost concluded that autistic children, (1) related to objects, (2) did not relate to their peers, (3) were unable to accept changes in routine, and (4) showed minimum affection for adults and avoided physical contact.

Autistic children often direct clear and articulate speech to certain individuals, while to others they are "elective mutes" (Morris, 1953). Mutism is a sort of protective barrier erected against a hostile environment.

Theoretical Interpretations

There is hardly a more controversial clinical concept than autism. It seems that practically every neurologist, psychiatrist, and psychologist who works with disturbed children has developed his own theory concerning autism. The relevant literature goes into hundreds of thousands of printed pages.

Certainly the term autism can be used for the description of a single symptom. Aloofness, withdrawal, speech disorder, and limited contact with reality can accompany a variety of organic and nonorganic mental disorders. But this terminological ambiguity applies to a variety of psychopathological concepts. Consider, for example, depression. Depression is a name of a symptom that accompanies most neuroses and psychoses; depression is the subjective feeling created by assaults of the superego upon the ego. It is a symptom of a self-directed aggression. However, the term depression is often used as a name of the affective or manic-depressive psychosis (see Wittenborn, 1965).

I use the terms autism, infantile autisms, and autistic schizophrenia as synonymous, to describe a severe syndrome of infantile schizophrenia. Thus, the following discussion will be limited to certain theoretical interpretations of this particular syndrome.

I believe that autism is a withdrawal mechanism. The archaic ego, barely formed in the first year of life, withdraws from contact with the outer world, which does not supply supportive libido cathexes. Autism is morbid, but it is a *morbid adjustment* for survival. The child blocks out emotions and withdraws from social contact. He fears people, for any contacts he has had have been painful and horrifying. Whenever mother gave milk, she scolded; when the infant called for help, mother got furious; whenever he cried at night, mother and father got mad (cf. Rimland, 1964).

No child is born autistic. Autism is a part of the schizophrenic downward adjustment; it is a withdrawal in order to avoid further damage (Nagelberg et al., 1953). The child is overwhelmed by hostile attitudes and has no alternative but to surrender; there is no use to fight against mother. The autistic child is a child who has given up growth, desire, initiative, emotions, and social contacts in order to survive. When it is impossible to get approval for one's actions, inactivity is the only possible avenue of existence.

Garcia and Sarvis (1964) believe that autism is a useful reaction to overwhelming assaults at a vulnerable developmental stage of six to 18 months, when the infant is just beginning to differentiate himself from his mother. The autistic infant feels that mother is persecuting him, and he rejects her by assuming a *basic paranoid* attitude. If the mother meets the reaction by a counterrejection, the infant's paranoid attitude will persist and develop into autism.

Garcia and Sarvis believe that autism is a reaction to multiple etiological agents "operating as gradients in any combination with each other and at varying levels of intensity and duration." In a case of a $3\frac{1}{2}$ year old boy they found a combination of inborn hyperreactivity, probable neurological damage, and the birth of a sister. The mother denied any pathology in the infant, and the father's enjoyment of the child's outbursts reinforced the autistic behavior. According to Garcia and Sarvis, autism is a reaction of the primitive ego to family psychopathology. For lack of available defenses the immature ego withdraws from contact with the outer world. Magical and delusionary thought processes, decline in motor skills and speech, and lack of relations with the environment are the main autistic symptoms.

Autistic children frequently display preference for olfactory contact with the environment. One can see these children smelling and sniffing and touching objects with their noses. Goldfarb (1956) noticed their preference for "contact receptors" such as smell, touch, and taste and avoidance of "distant receptors" such as sight and hearing. This regression to lower sensory contacts seems to fall in line with the over-all trend of adjustment for survival on a lower level of functioning.

Mahler (1952) distinguished two types of infantile psychosis: *autistic* and *symbiotic*. In the first type, the mother "never seems to have been perceived emotionally by the infant, and the first representation of outer reality, the mother as a person, as a separate entity, seems not to be cathected. The mother remains a part object seemingly devoid of specific cathexis and not distinguished from inanimate objects" (1952, p. 289). "The instinctual forces, both libido and aggression, exist in an unneutralized form, due to the absence of the synthetic function of the ego. There is an inherent lack of contact with the human environment."

Early infantile autism develops when the infant "devoid of emotional ties to the person of the mother is unable to cope with external stimuli and inner excitations, which threaten from both sides his very existence as an entity. Autism is, therefore, a mechanism by which such patients try to shut out, to hallucinate away (negative hallucination) the potential sources of sensory perception, particularly those which demand affective response. . . . The most striking feature is their spectacular struggle against any demand of human (social) contact which might interfere with their hallucinatory delusional need to command a static, greatly constricted segment of their inanimate environment in which they behave like omnipotent magicians. . . . These patients experience outer reality as an intolerable source of irritation, without specific or further qualification" (Mahler, 1952, p. 297).

Mahler believes that the autistic disorder is "the basic defense attitude of these infants for whom the beacon of emotional orientation in the outer world—the mother as primary love objects—is non-existent" (*ibid.*, p. 297).

Mahler and Gosliner (1955) established the period of 12-18 to 36 months of age, called the separation-individuation phase of personality, as being crucial for the ego and the development of object relationships (1955, p. 196). In 1958 Mahler continued her analysis of the development of autism. According to Mahler there are two main interlocked factors, namely, "Atrophy of the instinct of self-preservation and immaturity of apparatuses at birth" (Mahler, 1955, p. 77). Autism is a product of the failure of emergence of or return to the first two developmental stages of undifferentiated early mother-child unity. "'Some catastrophic shifts and reactions seem to be the pathogenic agents in early infant autism" (*ibid.*, p. 78). Autistic infants seem to have failed to emerge from the extra-uterine stage and are unable to develop normally.

In 1968 Mahler came out with a further elaboration of her theory. All neonates are autistic and cannot distinguish their own tension-reducing attempts from mother's soothing help. Mother's holding behavior serves as "auxilliary" ego. At the ninth month the infant begins to separate from mother. Failure in mothering causes severe distress and prevents the perception of mother as being friendly and leads to autistic alienation.

I believe that autism is better interpreted by the theory of inter-individual cathexes. The infant's earliest object relationship is *instrumental*. A normal infant craves milk and love, but when in his first encounters with mother no love is given to him because his mother is also instrumental and stronger than the infant, the infant may be forced to give up his contacts with the outer world altogether.

Some infants fight, and they belong to the aretic type of childhood schizophrenia. Some do not defend themselves at all; they are the pseudo-amentive type. Some children lose the battle at its start and withdraw behind a protective shell. Whenever the battle is lost very early, autistic behavior dominates the picture. There is no evidence that any child is born with *early infantile autism* (cf. Chapter 5). Even the unusual early sensitivity in young children described by Bergman and Escalona (1949) was not innate; most probably these children were victims of mother's subtle, instrumental hostility disguised by pseudo-vectorialism.

My longitudinal studies and prolonged interviews with parents have made me rather suspicious of parental reports regarding early years of the patients. In practically all cases mothers suffer from guilt feelings and/or are afraid of the anticipated or previously experienced interviews with psychiatrists and psychologists. It is a proof of their well-entrenched schizogenic pattern of behavior to put all the blame on the child. The mothers present themselves as self-sacrificing martyrs who have given their lives for the poor child. This invariably pseudo-vectorial attitude that has been the single greatest pathogenic factor cannot suddenly disappear in the interview in the hospital. "Almost every mother," wrote Kanner, "recalled her astonishment at the child's failure to assume the usual anticipatory posture preparatory to being picked up. This kind of adjustment occurs universally at four months of age" (1960, p. 717). But these mothers did not tell Dr. Kanner what husbands, older siblings, and other relatives have told me in life-history-type interviews.

4. SYMBIOTIC SCHIZOPHRENIA

My hypothesis is that the formation of the ego is most seriously disturbed in the amentive and autistic childhood schizophrenics. The neonate has no ego. His entire mental apparatus consists of the id, "a cauldron of seething excitement." "Within the id," wrote Freud, "the organic *instincts* operate, which are themselves composed of fusions of two primal forces (Eros and destructiveness). . . . The one and only endeavor of these instincts is toward satisfaction. But an immediate and regardless satisfaction of instinct, such as the id demands, would often enough lead to perilous conflicts with the external world and to extinction." "The other agency of the mind . . . the ego was developed out of the cortical layer of the id. . . . Its constructive function consists in interposing between the demand made by an instinct and the action that satisfies it, an intellective activity which . . . endeavors by means of experimental actions to calculate the consequences of the proposed line of conduct . . . just as the id is directed exclusively to obtaining pleasure, so the ego is governed by considerations of safety. The ego has set itself the task of self-preservation which the id appears to neglect. . . . In its efforts to preserve itself in an environment of overwhelming mechanical forces, the ego is threatened by dangers that come in the first instance from external reality, but not from there alone. Its own id is a source of similar dangers . . . an excessive strength of instinct can damage the ego in the same way as an excessive 'stimulus' from the external world. It is true that such an excess cannot destroy it; but it *can* destroy its characteristic dynamic organization, it can turn the ego back into a portion of id." (Freud, 1949, pp. 108-111.)

The weak, immature, "archaic" ego of the first phase of childhood becomes a storage of self-cathected libido. "We call this state of things absolute, primary *narcissism*. It continues until the ego begins to cathect the presentations of objects with libido—to change narcissistic libido into *object libido*. Throughout life the ego remains the great reservoir from which libidinal cathexes are sent out on to objects and into which they are also once more withdrawn. . . . It is only when someone is completely in love that the main quantity of libido is transferred onto the object and the object to some extent takes the place of the ego" (*ibid.*, pp. 23-24).

Sometimes "the weak and immature ego of the first phase of childhood is permanently damaged by the strain put upon it in the effort to ward off the dangers that are peculiar to that period of life. Children are protected against the dangers threatening them from the external world by the care of their parents; they pay for their security by a fear of losing their parents' love, which would deliver them over helpless to the dangers of the external world" (*ibid.*, p. 112).

This is precisely what happens in childhood schizophrenics. When the newborn is offered no protection, when he is exposed to violent scenes, verbal and nonverbal, *his ego may not emerge from the id and not become a libido-cathected, separate entity.* This is probably the situation in the pseudo-amentive schizophrenic. However, should the situation become less harsh, an emergence of the ego may still be possible.

When in the first months some protection is offered to the infant accompanied with great stress and instrumental demands, his weak, just-emerging ego may regress. It is no longer primary narcissism, for his infantile ego has already rushed to cathect his mother. In a self-protective move, the ego shuns contacts with anybody and anything. This is autistic withdrawal and regression of the infantile ego.

Some schizophrenic mothers are rejecting-protective, some are symbiotic-parasitic. Children of the latter group of mothers receive more support than the children of the rejecting-protective parents. Their mothers are somehow more willing to give affection to the child; they are not so harsh, though they are not less dictatorial. They are, indeed, unable to give. But *when they perceive the child as a part of themselves, giving away becomes giving to oneself.*

In symbiotic childhood schizophrenia this is precisely the situation. Mothers of symbiotic schizophrenic children are less hostile and more symbiotic-parasitic. They protect the child and "invade" his personality. Many adult manifest schizophrenics were symbiotic as infants. One of my patients, a 24 year old man, had been spoon fed and kept home for weeks in bad weather. Many catatonics were symbiotic schizophrenics in infancy. Their mothers conquered the child as one conquers a foreign territory and claims an absolute possession. They subjugated the child to their own emotional needs and prevented his normal growth. Yet their attitude was less destructive than the attitude of the rejecting-protective mothers of the pseudo-amentive and autistic children.

In terms of personality dynamics, a symbiotic childhood schizophrenia is caused by a *premature, precocious formation of an over-demanding, dictatorial, primitive superego.* In the pseudo-amentive syndrome no opportunity for growth has been given. In the autistic syndrome the only way to survive is to stay away from unbearable reality and regress into the dream world of unconscious. The archaic ego has renounced reality and again become "a portion of the id." A similar process takes place in hebephrenic and simple deterioration types of adult schizophrenics. In the symbiotic childhood schizophrenia, the child identifies with the mother by introjection of her image and renounces his own identity. He ceases to be a separate individual.

The symbiotic, subservient pattern of living in which the child renounces his independence, his strivings, and ambitions, even his pain and pleasure, seems to be the only way to secure his mother's love, to protect her, and as a result, his own life. The schizophrenic paradox of giving up everything to protect those who are supposed to be protectors is the leading motive in symbiotic schizophrenia (Wolman, 1957; 1966a; Mahler, 1958, 1968). It is the typical schizophrenic pattern of morbid downward adjustment for survival. "These mothers," wrote Hill, "are devastatingly, possessively, all-loving of their child who is to become schizophrenic . . . the condition for their love is one which the schizophrenic child cannot meet. If he does, to a degree, meet it, in so doing, he sacrifices his realization of a personality of his own, independent of hers" (Hill, 1955, p. 109).

Mothers of symbiotic children are anxiously possessive, affectionately overprotective, and jealously preventive of normal contacts between the child and the outer world. They keep the child home when the weather is bad, when the sun is too bright, when dogs are around. They prevent the child from playing with other children because of germs, measles, and other contagious diseases. They do everything for the child instead of letting the child do things for himself because the child may spill milk or break a cup and hurt himself.

This maternal symbiotic attitude forces *the formation of the superego prior to an adequate formation of the ego*. Normally, part of the ego develops into superego in the Oedipal conflict. In these children, the superego starts at the anal or perhaps even oral stage. The precociously formed superego takes over and distorts reality testing; although the child may have good mental abilities and use them properly in certain areas, he is anxious to give the "right answer," i.e., the answer that pleases his mother. A therapist once asked a preschool child: "Do you like these blue booklets?" The child's reply was: "Mommy says blue is a nice color."

The precocious formation of superego leads to hallucinated feelings of superparental power. Schizophrenic hallucinations are hallucinations of power, of omniscience and omnipotence. World saving and world destruction are frequent themes of schizophrenic delusions and hallucination. A schizophrenic, who has lost his grip on reality, may imagine himself as being capable of taking care of or destroying his parents. He "takes the law in his hands," as one patient put it, or he tries to control the world and shape its order.

In the symbiotic syndrome the child identifies with his mother too much and too early. The internalized mother image prevents further growth, other identifications, and independent thought or action. The child's perception of the world is highly distorted; he avoids other children and cannot relate to them; all his thoughts and feelings go out to his mother.

With this overidentification with his mother, separation must represent a terrible threat. The moods of a symbiotic child resemble the adult catatonic and are guided by a constant effort to keep his mother, to be with her, to please her, to do what she wants. The child has no initiative of his own, no interest, no ambitions to be fulfilled.

The Symbiotic Bond

A description of a case follows:

When Johnny came with his mother, he held on to her and refused to leave her hand. He followed her everywhere; when she sat down, he stood next to her chair. She sat down with a sigh and a moan. She was a heavy, talkative, verbose woman, and described in great detail her troubles with her husband and son. She was the self-sacrificing martyr who had married a "selfish, inconsiderate man" and had had with him this "poor, mentally retarded child."

Johnny was six years old, pale and obese. He pulled her hand and interrupted her speech with questions not related to mother's story. His speech was blurred; he swallowed syllables, and his voice did not carry well. He was definitely overdressed; he wore three sweaters. According to mother, Johnny was susceptible to common colds.

Whenever a question was directed to Johnny, his mother answered for him. She was vehemently hostile to her husband but not overtly hostile to her child. To the contrary, during the session, she hugged and kissed Johnny, and whenever she burst out in tears, her affection for Johnny seemed to grow.

Johnny cried together with his mother, although one could not be sure whether he was really moved by the content of her story. Most probably he automatically responded to her tears irrespective of their cause and with little attention to the content of her story.

Johnny had no friends nor playmates. On weekends mother took him to the park, but she never allowed him to play with other children because "they were dirty," and Johnny was a "sensitive child" and easily caught diseases. No child was allowed to visit Johnny's home; nor was Johnny allowed to visit other children. The reason given by the mother was the

danger of infectious diseases and her conviction that Johnny was unable
to defend himself against other children who (all of them) are aggressive.

Johnny liked dogs but his mother seemed to be jealous even of animal
friends. Her excuse was that dogs bite and have fleas and poor Johnny
might get bitten by dogs and fleas.

In reply to my question, the mother maintained that she wished Johnny
to become more outgoing and independent. At this moment Johnny
asked her to tie his shoelaces. She refused. Johnny repeated his demand;
he raised his voice and screamed.

His mother called him "monster," but yielded to his whim and tied the
laces. I imagine that such battles have occurred daily. Johnny was
taught to rely on his mother in everything; he was repeatedly told how
incompetent and inadequate he was. He was discouraged from doing
anything on his own; whenever he dared to try, he was criticized for his
clumsiness. Gradually he gave up trying. *The only way to please mother
was to depend on her* and make her believe that she was an indispensable,
generous, and most kind person. Johnny was afraid to alienate his mother
and ceased to live his own life. He somehow knew that he was expected
to ask mother's help in everything. Though occasionally his mother
protested, her anger was at a minimum as compared with her malicious,
venomous criticism whenever Johnny dared to do anything on his own
without referring to his mother.

I once tested a 19 year old schizophrenic who, I believe, was a
classic case of an "overstayed" infantile symbiotic schizophrenia.
His mother was still helping him to dress in the morning; she put
cream and sugar in his coffee and helped him to get ready for college. She took care of his classroom notebooks; she helped him to
write papers; she typed and retyped them; she kept records of his
tests and marks. She invited "company" home for him, but he himself had no boy or girl friends. He was afraid to contradict his
mother, but once in a while he burst out in a fury, cursed, and even
hit his mother. His father was rarely home; occasionally he was
present but a nonparticipating observer.

Another patient, a 17 year old girl belonged to the same category.
Her mother washed her hair, took her out, fed her, and did not
allow her to associate with anyone else.

A symbiotic child, as it were, becomes a part of his mother. He
repeats what his mother says; he tries to read her mind and to be
the way he feels she wants him to be. He follows her wherever she
goes, showers her with questions to make sure his thoughts follow
hers. He cannot share her with anyone else, for his security depends

on a religious adherence to his mother, to fixed rules, and to definite schedules. The slightest deviation from routine and the mildest frustration throws the child into a state of panic and unleashes a catatonic-type hostility.

To symbiotic overidentification with the mother, separation must represent a terrible threat. The moods of a symbiotic child resemble those of the adult catatonic. They are guided by a constant effort to keep his mother, to be with her, to please her, to do what she wants. The child renounces initiative of his own and shows no interest, no ambitions to be fulfilled.

Hostility

Schizophrenia in adults is associated with a continuous effort to control pent-up hostility. Normal children are often angry at their parents, but schizophrenic children are angry at themselves for being angry at their parents. Parents of schizophrenic children present themselves to their children as weak, unhappy martyrs; who can be angry at them?

An 11 year old schizophrenic girl was savagely beaten by her father. According to the father's story she was his "nice little girl," until she dared to reject his amorous "affection." According to the girl's story, her father was a former "great opera singer" (which he never had been), persecuted by powerful and malicious enemies, misunderstood by his wife, and suffering from a severe heart condition. His heart condition was one of the family myths. He was an ex-third-rate cabaret singer, currently a hotel clerk whose personal life was far from making him a paragon of morality.

When the father "punished" the girl for talking to boys in the street, the girl took the beating patiently. Her only worry was that her father might hurt his hand or overexert himself and get a heart attack.

Her anger and hurt feelings were repressed, but the lid went off a few days later. The girl was overinvolved with her "poor" mother, and could not do anything without mother's permission and her active participation. On that evening, the girl, who had no friends, asked her mother to "take her" to the movies. The mother was busy and answered impatiently, "It is just three blocks away! A girl your age can go by herself! And, by the way, why don't you have friends?"

The girl flared up. She believed that her symbiotic behavior was a sign of her loyalty and devotion, and here her mother "rejected" her. The girl grabbed a bottle of Coca-Cola and threw it at her mother. She missed the mother; she maintained that she had missed intentionally, but could not control her pent-up hostility.

A five year old boy tore up mother's skirt and kicked her vehemently when she told him that he must go to kindergarten. Symbiotic children become entangled by their mothers, but once they are entangled they cannot disentangle themselves. Any effort to loosen the tie throws the child into a state of panic and fury. His fury resembles catatonia—it is directed against everything and everybody including himself.

Theoretical Interpretations

An interesting theory of symbiosis was proposed by Mahler based on intensive research and devoted therapeutic work with schizophrenic children. According to Mahler (1952, 1955) during the first 12 to 18 months the infant is "an almost completely vegetative being symbiotically dependent on the mother" (Mahler and Gosliner, 1955, p. 195). Then a period of "individuation-separation" or "hatching from the symbiotic-mother child common membrane" starts. Mahler, being influenced by M. Klein, interprets the symbiotic child psychosis as a failure of separation-individuation of the ego. Normally, the first 12 to 18 months are "symbiotic." Then, from 18 to 36 months a separation-individuation process takes place (Mahler and Gosliner, 1955). If the symbiotic phase has been adequate, the child enters the next phase.

The mechanisms of the symbiotic psychosis are "introjective-projective," said Mahler, which aim at a "restoration of the symbiotic parasitic delusion of oneness with the mother and thus are the diametric opposites of the function of autism . . . clinical symptoms manifest themselves between the ages of two and a half to five, with a peak of onset in the fourth year of life. There infants' reality ties depend mainly upon the delusional fusion with the mother unlike those of the autistic who had no reality ties to begin with" (Mahler, 1952, p. 297-298).

Mahler believes that symbiotic-psychotic children are constitutionally vulnerable. "The very existence of the constitutional ego defect in the child . . . helps create the vicious circle . . . by stimulating mother to react to the child in an overanxious way" (1955, p. 201).

I see no reason to postulate "constitutional ego defects." It seems methodologically preferable to assume that the id is the constitutional part of personality and that both ego and superego develop in interaction in the family. Some little patients in the Sonia Shankman Orthogenic School (Bettelheim, 1950) compared the counselor to their own parents: parents love, counselors "becare." Love meant to these children a demanding attitude, "becare" was giving, was vectorial. The parents of schizophrenic children either do not love at all and demand love from their children, as most of the fathers do, or love the child but demand too much in return, as the mothers do (see Chapter 3). The schizophrenic child learns that strings are always attached to parental love. The schizophrenic child has been told that he does not deserve parental love. This is said day by day and several times each day of his life. In order to win love, he must be perfect.

Some children develop obsessive-compulsive symptoms to ward off their own "bad" inclinations: this schizo-type neurosis will be described in Chapter 4. Some children, as it were, make a halfway adjustment and compromise and develop schizoid character neurosis. Some children keep desperately struggling against their being "bad"; these are the latent schizophrenics. Some of these children break the symbiotic bond and develop aggressive behavioral patterns somewhat resembling those of psychopaths.

This belligerent type of childhood schizophrenia has been named *aretic*.

5. THE ARETIC SYNDROME*

Some infants display unusual aggressiveness and unprovoked cruelty. Once a five year old boy was brought to my office after he had almost strangled his little play companion to death. His previous experiences had been biting his two year old sister and hitting a playmate with a heavy stick. Some infants bite, scratch, tear hair, and badly hurt other children. They also hurt themselves by scratching their own faces, pulling their hair, banging their heads, etc. Boatman and Szurek (1960) in their comprehensive study of childhood schizophrenics reported a girl who hit the head of another girl against a concrete wall and a four year old girl who deliberately

---

* The term "aretic" means belligerent. It is derived from Ares, the Greek god of war.

slammed the door on her own finger. In a children's ward in one of the hospitals where I worked, there were children who were almost completely bald after they had torn out most of their hair; some of them swallowed the hair. Many children had to be psysically restrained from causing serious physical harm to themselves and to others.

I interviewed the parents of these children. All of them were exasperated and bewildered by the child's aggressive and self-aggressive behavior. The parents blamed one another for "spoiling" the child and for pathological heredity, being unaware of their peculiar interaction with each other and with their child.

Some infants were literally crushed by parental anxieties, moods, and outbursts of hostility that accompanied an unwilling but nevertheless dutiful care. The growth of these children was inhibited and frozen into a *pseudo-amentive* vegetation. Other infants who had received a little more maternal warmth began to grow and blossom, but soon the mother's angry and demanding impatience and/or the father's indifference or brutality forced them to withdraw into an *autistic* protective shell. Still other infants had received more warmth and affection, but their mothers had demanded a high price for their limited love and insisted on unlimited submission to their whims. The child received maternal love only when he agreed to surrender his own personality and accept a *symbiotic-submissive* tie with his mother.

An *aretic* schizophrenic is a child who receives, in his first year or two, sufficient affection to enable some initial ego growth, but not enough to control his resentment against the instrumental robbing mother. The child would like to please his mother and to protect her when she claims he makes her sick. He would like to be her quiet, nice, little child, and he does enjoy occasional bits of the high-priced parental approval. The aretic child may even have some development of superego, resulting from an initial identification with one of the parents. Yet he is unable to renounce his will entirely and fights against a complete surrender. His ego is not strong enough to accept frustration and control his resentment, nor can he believe anymore that his mother is always right, always good and kind as she professes to be. The aretic child has had sufficient mental growth to enable him to realize how unfair, demanding, and selfish is his mother. He carries the image of the *bad mother* who cares but hurts, who gives a little and demands a lot in return. This feeling that mother is bad, makes the child angry at his mother and angry at himself for hating his mother.

Ambivalence

Aretic children are symbiotic but rebellious. They cling to their parents, yet attack them. They resent being left alone even for a while, yet they do not seem to enjoy proximity with their parents. Aretic children are torn by ambivalent feelings toward their parents, typical of adult schizophrenics who hate themselves for hating their overdemanding parents. Aretic children are intensely involved with their parents, whom they love and hate at one and the same time. They wish they could change their parents and, with some magic trick, transform them into truly loving and kind individuals. An aretic child may say to his mother, "You are not a real Mommy; real mommies don't yell at their kids."

Yet a schizophrenic mother is sometimes nice to the child and does take care of him. She is a self-advertising hero who praises her self-sacrifice, but she does not abandon nor neglect the child. Aretic children that I saw in my private office and clinics were well fed, carefully clad, kept neat, and taken care of. The child is, in most cases, aware of mother's care and feels indebted to her, but her exaggerated demands and criticism make the child angry.

Seven year old Sharon threw a rock and broke a window pane in her parents suburban house. Then she cried and scratched her right hand badly as a punishment for breaking windows. She repeated in my office her mother's tirade, including a fantastic estimate of the cost of window panes. She felt sorry for her "poor" mother, and "poor" father, who indulged in oral sexual relations with his "nice little girl." Sharon pleased her father sexually because "he worked so hard and mommy fought with him," but she took out her resentment on her four year old brother and other children in the neighborhood, whom she terrorized.

Little Mary acted out her resentment directly against her mother. This four and a half year old girl went into tantrums whenever her mother left her home with the baby-sitter. Yet when the mother came back, the little girl would scream and hit and claw her. Boatman and Szurek (1960, p. 395) described some of these children as follows: "Even the child who clings to his parents usually does so in a possessively demanding and often physically hurtful way, showing little relaxation or enjoyment in contact with them. However indifferent or hurtful he is, particularly with his mother, he is clearly 'dependent' upon her and experiences panic on separation from her. We have seen somatic malfunction as an indirect manifestation of this struggle and panic, e.g., anorexia or bulimia, constipation or diarrhea, asthma and eczema."

The *dependence-independence* syndrome plays a most significant role in aretic childhood schizophrenia. The child rebels against being engulfed by his mother. He attacks her not only when in despair as a symbiotic child would do, but uses abusive language frequently and consciously, and physical force to test the results. The child seems to enjoy malicious, destructive, and hurtful deeds. He laughs when something is destroyed, obviously feeling his own power, power to disobey, to hurt, and to destroy. He may break his toys, tear his books, damage furniture, hit other children without necessarily being in a symbiotic panic or catatonic frenzy. Occasionally, $5\frac{1}{2}$ year old Tommy boasted of his deeds. Most probably he was testing: was he really a bad, dangerous person, a "killer," as his mother called him?

Punishment did not seem to have much restraining influence upon him. It rather increased his paranoid projections and introjections. When beaten by his father he knew for sure he was bad, mother was bad, and father was bad also. The world seemed to turn into a huge mass of hostility. The little boy fantasized and talked about killing, burning, and torturing. Occasionally, he acted out his aggressive fantasies.

Anality

Anal conflicts are of great significance in the development of all types of schizophrenia. At the time of toilet training the child learns "to postpone or to renounce a direct instinctual gratification out of consideration for the environment . . . but simultaneously the hitherto 'omnipotent' adult becomes dependent, to a certain degree, on the will of the child" (Fenichel, 1946, p. 278). The chances for a reversal of social age roles are greater than at any other stage, for this is the first time the parents *ask* the child to give them something that is the child's indisputable property—the feces.

At the time of the anal conflict some parents become exceedingly involved with the child. The child's resistance reawakens their own anxieties and makes them unhappy, angry, or both. The child cannot fail to notice how much his parents depend on him, that is, how weak they are. As a result, the child may experience elimination as an expression of a great self-sacrifice, for he gives up the pleasure of retention in order to please the demanding mother. Being insecure, schizophrenic mothers tend to appeal for sympathy and ask the infant to have pity on them. Under the threat of mother's self-advertised "martyrdom," the child gives away feces, his cherished possession. Once a mother described highly dramatic speeches, concerning bowel movements, that she delivered to her two and a half year old infant who later became a highly destructive schizophrenic child. The child renounces the cathexis of something which is in his body and overcathects his libido in an external object, the mother. Obviously, a similar though less extensive process may also take place in normal cases, but in schizophrenic children, toilet training is always severe and definitely *too* successful. Toilet training in schizophrenic children is accomplished with greatest perfection; the child surrenders pleasure to duty and develops compulsory cleanliness as a reaction formation to his desire to rebel and be dirty. In those cases where the ego can still control the outbursts of destrudo, the child will become a latent schizophrenic.

As a result of the anal conflict, the child may develop anal fears and phobias. He may fear that something wrong will happen to his parents should he fail them in the training for cleanliness. To be dirty means to them much more than it means to a normal person. They talk about cleanliness as if it were a moral duty or a religious commandment, and as if a violation of cleanliness were equal to a sacrilege.

By the same logic, any considerable neglect in external appearance in a latent schizophrenic carries a significant diagnostic and prognostic message, for it is one of the signs of the dangerous rebellion of the id. The ego seems to say: "I cannot take it any longer, and I do not care any more for my mother. Come what may, I will break loose." This rebellion increases the vitality of the individual, but it does not contribute to his ability to behave in a mentally nor-

mal manner. The aretic child is more active than an autistic or symbiotic one and his ego has attained a higher level of organization,
yet neither his ego nor superego is capable of exercising rational
control.

Anal fears play a significant role in the personality structure of
all schizophrenics. Psychoanalytic theory explains the nature of
these fears as follows: "As a retaliation for anal-sadistic tendencies,
fears develop for what one wished to perpetrate anally on others
will now happen to oneself. Fears of physical injury of an anal nature develop, like the fear of some violent ripping out of feces or
of body contents" (Fenichel, 1945, p. 68). In many cases of schizophrenic children, mothers had actually been forcefully "ripping
feces" out of the child's body by a forceful application of enemas
(cf. Fleck et al., 1959). The overanxious toilet training is perceived
by the child as a part of her over-all robbing attitude. The mother
takes away from the child his libido, his possessions, and even the
contents of his body. This is, I believe, the origin of ideas of reference in schizophrenics who believe that some people steal their
thoughts.

Schizogenic mothers and fathers use their child to satisfy their
own emotional needs. The aretic child is a child who has not
had the chance to rationalize, to displace, or to develop other
defense mechanisms. He has faced the alternative of a complete
subservience to the mother or an overt rebellion of impulses. As
in all other types of schizophrenics, the choice is between the superego or id, with the ego crushed in between.

Bender (1959) observed pseudo-psychopathic symptoms in
schizophrenic children. Some of them steal, lie, assault people, and
destroy property, and many of them are "children who hate" (Redl
and Wineman, 1960). Undoubtedly, many delinquent children and
adults are schizophrenic.

There is, however, a profound difference between aggressive psychopaths and those schizophrenic children who become aggressive.
Psychopaths attack for gains. They are hyperinstrumental and steal
money to use it; they attack others to force their submission and
they steal toys or money. They are, so to speak, practical delinquents, who fight for material gains or for self-assertion and control
of others. Psychopaths (hyperinstrumentals) believe they are right
in attacking others. They avoid fights with anyone who can retaliate

or fight them off, and they usually attack weak subjects; their hostility is the wolf versus sheep type (see Chapter One).

A schizophrenic aggressor is a child who has failed to control his hostility toward his parents. He is a child tortured by guilt feelings whenever he attacks others and who wishes to be restrained. Yet he is often carried away and unable to control his impulses. If he steals, his thefts are senseless; he attacks people who are stronger than himself; he assaults foe and friend alike, and exposes himself to terrible retaliation. His hostile, destructive acts may be acts of compulsion combined with *paranoid hallucination,* though the violent acts of aretic children resemble senseless hebephrenic-type destructiveness with hallucinations of grandeur. The aretic child fights against "bad people," because he was told (and believed that it was true) that he himself is a "bad boy." He projects self-accusations by blaming others and, with the typical, infantile-psychotic lack of self-restraint, attacks everyone.

The Bad-Me

A five year old girl was senselessly destructive in kindergarten. When intercepted, she whispered that she was "the bad fairy." The acceptance of being bad is one of the most significant differences between paranoid and hebephrenic schizophrenics. Paranoids project hostility—hebephrenics, as a rule, do not; rather they introject.

In childhood, such as transition is quite easy. The child's perception of himself and of his mother is crucial for the development of his ego and superego, respectively. In hypervectorial children the perception of oneself is subordinated to the perception of mother and to what the child thinks of his mother's attitude toward himself. Hence, there are fluctuations between projection and introjection.

Normally, the protective parental attitude enables the infant to develop the self-protective apparatus, the ego. When the parents are not protective, no ego can develop, as is the case in the pseudoamentive schizophrenic. Very little if any ego develops in the autistic and symbiotic schizophrenics. In all these cases, the ego either does not develop at all or it regresses and merges again with the id. The lack of ego or "no-ego" is perceived or experienced by the individual *as not being himself* and being exposed to a mortal danger without any protection whatsoever. This feeling corresponds to Sullivan's *"not-me"* (cf. Sullivan, 1947, 1953, 1962). This is a weird, uncanny feeling frequently experienced in the autistic and symbiotic types of infantile schizophrenia. Symbiotic schizophrenics experience this feeling whenever separated from mother; adult schizophrenics experience it in precipitous psychotic breakdown (cf. Hill, 1955). Manifest schizophrenics feel "not-me" whenever their ego loses all vestige of control and seems to disappear.

The feeling *"bad-me"* borrowed from Sullivan, is a description of *surrender of the ego to the superego*. The reader is reminded of our emphatic distinction between the milder paranoid and catatonic syndromes of manifest schizophrenia in which the ego surrenders to superego, the more severe hebephrenia where id is victorious, and the most severe simple deterioration where the organism seems to give up life altogether (see Chapter 1).

The same distinction applies to schizophrenia in childhood. In aretic schizophrenia the child's perception of self is not "not-me," but "bad-me." (cf. Sullivan, 1947, 1962). The "bad me" feeling is a complex product of perceiving mother as a potential enemy, introjection of her image, and identification with her.

A normal child may occasionally feel mother is unfair and express it. A normal mother brushes it off, and eventually picks up the child, consoles, and reassures. She tells him that she loves him and compensates for whatever wrong she has done to him. When the child feels reassured, he believes that his mother is good and protective and loves him, even if she occasionally scolds and disapproves of his behavior.

A schizogenic mother takes a child's resentment as a personal insult. She actually exploits the child's hostility for renewed attacks upon him. Mothers of aretic children blame the child even more for being a "bad child," "murderer of his own mother," etc. The aretic child finds himself enmeshed in a new double bind: mother who was the attacker turns into a victim, and he who was victimized becomes the bad child. A symbiotic child yields, renounces his ego, his identity. The aretic child hates; he hates himself, and even more hates mother. He knows that he is bad, and his mother is bad too. A four and a half year old boy who hit another child with a hoe over the head said, "I don't care if he dies." Yet when he hurt his mother, he got panicky, became confused, and lost contact with reality. He hated himself for hating his mother. His weak ego could not take it and he felt this time "not-me."

CHAPTER 4

Schizophrenia in Later Childhood and Adolescence

1. UPS AND DOWNS

Growing up is not always growing out. Without a planned therapeutic or an unplanned compensatory interaction, the psychotic child may get worse as he grows up. In some cases, a friendly relative or neighbor or teacher may offer the sick child encouragement and emotional support. Such a supportive relationship may improve the balance of cathexes and enable compensatory development of the child's ego, but not all schizophrenic children are fortunate. Many of them drop out of school after failing in scholastic and social adjustment; some are placed in schools and institutions for the mentally retarded, while others have never attended school because their parents have been much too embarrassed and kept the children home. I worked with a 10 year old boy whose parents took him out of the neighborhood public school and put him in a private school for mentally retarded despite the boy's normal I.Q. Another child's annoying and destructive behavior was used by his parents as an excuse for placing him in a boarding home for mentally retarded children.

Schizophrenic children present a gloomy clinical picture of pseudo-amentive, autistic, symbiotic, and aretic schizophrenia. Some symptoms look milder as the children grow up, yet most schizophrenic children of school age still have difficulties with eating, sleeping, speech, personal care, and sometimes even bowel and bladder control. Schizophrenic children are torn by unbearable anxieties or given to uncontrollable impulses, creating additional difficulties for their not too well adjusted parents. Most schizophrenic children are disruptive in classrooms, and only some of them can somehow relate to their peers (cf. Bettelheim, 1950; Geleerd, 1946).

109

The great variety of schizophrenic symptoms in childhood defeats all efforts at classification. All children grow physically and mentally, whether their growth is good or poor, and a 12 year old child with an I.Q. of 25 is quite different from a normal three year old child, despite the fact that their mental age is equal. The 12 year old child is not a three year old, no matter how poor his development has been.

The same holds true in regard to schizophrenics. The pseudo-amentive, autistic, symbiotic, and aretic children grow up. They have more and new experiences, many of them learn to talk, and all of them somehow perceive the environment and relate to it. All of them are exposed to pleasurable and painful stimuli, get sick and well, and live among other people. None of them remains fixated and unchanged.

Some of them move up; some go down. In the Mental Hygiene Clinic where I worked for many years I saw children who reportedly had been pseudo-amentive and autistic in the first two or three years of their lives, but later went to school where they experienced not too serious academic difficulties. On the other hand, I saw a great many children who badly deteriorated within a few years. Prognosis in childhood schizophrenics is, to even greater extent than in the adult schizophrenic, a matter of not who is the patient, but *who will take care* of him (see Chapter 7).

Prediction in schizophreno-type disorders always hinges on patterns of social interaction. Kris reported longitudinal child development studies conducted by the Child Study Center of the Yale University School of Medicine (1957). In one case, on the basis of Rorschach and interviews with a pregnant mother, the research workers predicted an early and overstrict toilet training. Observing the child in her third year of life, the investigators found that the child could not bear to see the tiniest spot of dirt on her dress. Her mother was, however, rather inconsistent in her efforts, and when the little girl reached her fourth birthday, she was not yet toilet trained. The research workers concluded that they could not foresee the real incidents that life brings along, such as birth of a sibling, the attitude of siblings, teachers, schoolmates, separation or death of parents, death of grandparents, etc.

Apparently, these *real incidents represent the crucial interactional factors that determine whether schizophrenia will develop, to what degree, what kind of syndromes, etc.* Sociogenic factors of power and acceptance and interindividual cathexis do and undo mental disorders (cf. Chapter 1), and one's mental health improves and deteriorates depending on how and who interacts with him (Wolman, 1970a).

There has been a noticeable tendency to include under the name childhood schizophrenia any atypical or bizarre behavioral pattern. As will be explained in Chapter 7, classification on the basis of mere symptomatology does not serve any useful purpose. Criticism against overinclusion has been raised by several workers (Despert and Sherwin, 1958; Kanner and Eisenberg, 1955; and others).

For practical purposes I would suggest dividing all hypervectorial (schizo-type) school-age disorders into three groups, namely, manifest psychotic, latent psychotic, and neurotic. Schizophrenia is not a static defect, but a changing process with ups and downs, especially in childhood, where there is a natural process of growth and an incessant contact with the family environment. In contradistinction to adult schizophenics, schizophrenic children are children subject to the maturational process that in normal conditions leads through the developmental stages of emotional, intellectual, and over-all personality growth. Children are continuously exposed to conditioning and cathexis through their contacts with parents, siblings, teachers, and peers. While some parts of their personality can be badly affected by this social interaction, other parts may keep growing. All this results in intriguing discrepancies in the schizophrenic child and in astonishing intraindividual differences of intellectual and social behavior in the same child that makes one wonder how can such mutually contradictory personality traits and behavioral patterns coexist in one individual.

2. MANIFEST CHILDHOOD SCHIZOPHRENIA

In view of what has been said I shall not try to trace in children the four types of adult schizophrenia, but seek instead the most common symptoms and interpret them. I agree with the definition offered by Boatman and Szurek (1960, p. 394): "We consider a child to be psychotic when his disorder is so great that almost all affective expression is distorted and when, in addition, his capacity to experience real satisfaction and to learn at his age level is seriously interferred with."

The symptoms of adult schizophrenics (see Chapter 1) include an over-all decline of vitality, lowered resistance to illness, disbalance in sleep and in the intake of food, and neglect of personal cleanliness. The cognitive functions in schizophrenia are highly disturbed by the invasion of primary processes with prelogical way of thinking, delusions, and hallucinations. Their moods are usually depressed, and self-esteem is practically nonexistent. Their social life oscillates between overinvolvement and withdrawal, accompanied by inevitable frustrations and a profound feeling of loneliness. The extreme object hypercathexis and resulting impoverishment of self-cathexis create a feeling of emptiness, of not being oneself, and depersonalization. Adult manifest schizophrenics failed to develop a clear-cut sexual identification, and they have not sublimated their sexual and hostile impulses. As a result of psychological changes, psychosomatic symptoms have developed.

In contradistinction to some other workers, I believe that childhood schizophrenia is not a separate clinical entity but one of the patterns of the great group of schizophrenias, the *vectoriasis praecox*. All of the symptoms of the manifest adult schizophrenic are, with some modifications, also found in childhood schizophrenics.

The clinical picture of childhood schizophrenia is complicated. I treated a 10 year old boy who started as a pseudo-amentive, but who received some degree of approval and affection later in life, yet not enough to develop an adequate ego; he began to talk at the age of three, but became symbiotically overattached not to his mother but to a friendly aunt who acted as a mother substitute. When he had reached the age of 10, he did not function at the full level of his intellectual capacity, but he was not pseudo-amentive; he developed a symbiotic attachment and was compliant, but he had frequent rebellious outbursts and tantrums. He perspired profusely, and his homeostasis was inadequate; he had serious social difficulties, but he was not autistic nor symbiotic. The difficulty in classification of manifest psychotic children stems from the fact that schizophrenia is not a static defect but a dynamic, multiphasic process. Combined with natural growth and learning in childhood, this disorder gives a multiplicity of behavioral patterns, largely depending upon each individual's life history.

The behavioral differences should be traced to the origins of the disorder (pseudo-amentive, autistic, symbiotic, aretic, and neurotic), to later developments in life with their ups and downs, and to the patterns of interaction with the child's environment. The importance of this continuous healing or hurting interaction can be hardly overestimated. Its impact through cathexis or conditioning or both was explained in Chapter 1 and will be restated in several other places in this volume.

The discussion of the etiology of schizophrenia was presented in Chapter 2. If childhood schizophrenia is a sociogenic disorder, it is certainly not a product of a single traumatic experience. It is highly improbable that it could start as late as in the school years after a perfectly normal childhood. In about 30 years of clinical experience in hospitals, clinics, and in private office setting, I have never seen any schizophrenic, child or adult, whose first five or six years were reasonably normal. A review of the research literature shows that such a thing is hardly possible. A normal child at the beginning of the latency period is not as dependent at this period on parental moods as schizophrenic children are. Suppose the parents who have acted normally for six years have suddenly changed, or that the child is placed with foster parents who hate one another. Certainly the child will suffer, but it is doubtful whether a normal child will develop at the latency period a vehement object hypercathexis with an impoverishment of self-cathexis, with an overgrowth of superego and other elements of *vectoriasis praecox*. The professional literature describes several cases where a peculiar type of a trauma was described as the onset of manifest schizophrenia. I have seen cases where a disease or an accident or death of the father or of a paternal substitute was the starting point of a psychotic breakdown or of a rapid psychotic deterioration. In all these cases, the peculiar trauma of loss or damage to the hypercathected love object was the precipitating factor. Perhaps it was more than the straw that broke the camel's back; it might have been a storm that destroyed a shack that was falling apart anyway. Schizophrenics cannot take loss of their hypercathected love objects.

There is a great deal of evidence (cf. Chapter 2) that childhood schizophrenia usually starts in the first year or first two years of life. If the harm is negligible or if the noxious schizogenic factors start later, the child develops not a manifest schizophrenia but a latent schizophrenia or a hypervectorial childhood neurosis. Later experiences determine whether his neurosis or latent psychosis will be arrested or improved, or whether a deterioration will occur. *A manifest schizophrenic child is a child in whom the ego either has not developed at all or has been badly damaged in his early years.* An adult manifest schizophrenic is either an "overstayed" case of childhood schizophrenia, or a person who has been in his childhood a latent schizophrenic or a hypervectorial neurotic who gradually or rapidly went through some or all five levels of deterioration (Wolman, 1966).

Main Symptoms

One of the most significant aspects of childhood schizophrenia is its extreme flexibility (Ekstein and Wallerstein, 1954). Perhaps flexibility is an understatement. The dictum "No one is schizophrenic all the time" applies to schizophrenic children even more than to adults. The processes of maturation and learning repeatedly offer new opportunities for improvement, if not recovery, and new ego compensatory symptoms are formed. A quiet harmonious atmosphere on weekends at home when father reads a newspaper and mother knits, or when the parents sit and converse in a friendly manner may give the child the feeling of security, increase his belief in parental power, and reduce the necessity to protect them by a lavish object cathexis. The child may for a while feel like a child. Should this peaceful coexistence continue or should there be a marked improvement in the interparental and parents-child relationship, some of the child's libido may become reinvested in himself and his ego may thrive anew (cf. Wolman, 1965a).

Most schizophrenic children show the lack of development and/or decline in personal care so typical of adult schizophrenics. In cases when an autistic child reaches school age and has not learned personal care, it is lack of development. In cases when a neurotic child deteriorates into psychosis, it is a decline. In either case, lack of personal cleanliness and care is a part of the downward adjustment that saves the energies of the impoverished organism. Passivity and apathy are the protective shell of exhaused or frightened organisms. An impoverished, inadequately self-cathected system is exceedingly prone to develop psychosomatic diseases, the allergies, common colds, skin troubles, and gastrointestinal and metabolic disorders so frequent in schizophrenic children.

Self-Awareness

One of the outstanding features of a schizophrenic child is his inability to experience a clear-cut perception of himself and his own identity. The child experiences no distinct limits to his boundaries and seems to merge with the objects in his environment. The term "dysidentity" describes the main problem, which is a distortion in the integration and appreciation of identities (Hendrickson, 1952). Other symptoms are secondary reactions to this basic dysidentity or disturbance in egofunctioning.

Schulman (1953) believes that childhood schizophrenia is the consequences of defective ego development which causes the child not to be able to cope with environmentally induced frustrations and to restrain unconscious impulses from disturbing thought processes. He feels that concept formation, "the level at which the schizophrenic child conceives of the relationship of environmental objects," is a measure of ego development (p. 11).

The child's ego begins to develop when he draws a line between himself and objects in his environment; the world begins to become real to the child when he sees himself in relation to things other than himself. A full recognition of the outer reality necessitates the use of concept formation.

Two factors influence the development of an inadequate concept formation in schizophrenic children. One is impairment in their thought development, and the other is their withdrawal and fear, both of which seem to be interrelated. As this process of withdrawal continues, the fear of extending thoughts beyond that which is considered "safe" increases. Thus the thought of schizophrenic children is narcissistic and autistic, and even those children who are of average intelligence or above have a difficult time acquiring *new* information and developing fresh concepts.

The fixation to infantile ways of thinking results in the absence of increase in the abstract conceptual ability with age. Apparently, most schizophrenic children are unable or fear to think beyond the well known as obvious.

Schizophrenic children exhibit impaired ability to perceive relationships. At practically all age levels they tend to use *concrete definitions* and cling to concrete aspects of objects. The "impaired ego in schizophrenic children prevents their adequately understanding the relationship of environmental objects" (Schulman, 1953, p. 15).

As early as in the first year the infant begins to realize that he has body boundaries and that his mother is a separate personality and a separate body in space. From that time on, through interaction with the environment, the child forms patterns of behavior and attitudes of mind related to his own developing ego (A. Freud, 1953; Owen, 1955; Spitz, 1965).

This development of self-awareness is delayed or uneven in schizophrenic children. A three year old schizophrenic child may not know where his body ends and the rest of the world begins. Schizophrenic children display impaired self-awareness, uncertainty about their own identity, and inability to distinguish clearly themselves from their environment (Goldfarb, 1961). Schizophrenic children show peculiar behavioral patterns, such as toe walking, rocking, and whirling, as if trying to test their own motor abilities.

Apparently, the schizophrenic child has no less difficulty in clarifying his ego boundaries, than he does his body boundaries (Soble, 1955; and others). Schizophrenic children have difficulty in identifying themselves and in relating to others, shifting from passive subservience to violent defiance.

When schizophrenic children examine things, they tend to overlook the objects as wholes and seem to perceive objects as if they were a series of details. They stress, on Rorschach inkblots, the little details and fail in generalizations (Piotrowski, 1945).

Many schizophrenic children exhibit body image disturbance and often perceive parts of their own bodies as foreign to themselves. In their human figure drawings, schizophrenic children often reveal distorted, omitted, or disproportional features or failure to link parts as a whole (Norman, 1954). On the Goodenough "Draw-a-Person" test, they reveal these mental disorganizations and others, such as disturbed spatial relationships, elongated parts, overemphasis on the extremities, and transparencies showing introjected bodies (Bakwin and Bakwin, 1960). Schizophrenic children reveal themes of gross mutilation and destruction or general bodily disintegration, and often dwell on the theme of death (Norman, 1954).

Goldfarb (1961), comparing schizophrenic and normal children, found no significant differences in physical characteristics and sensory apparatus. Schizophrenic children display more hyperactivity and hypoactivity than normal children. Schizophrenic children have difficulty in generalization, classification, and abstraction, and an inferior perception and conceptualization of time, space, and people.

Schizophrenic children develop many defensive behavioral patterns related to their inadequate time and space perception. Withdrawal, perseveration, insistence on sameness, confabulations, and compulsive overconcern with time and space seem to aim at reducing the child's anxiety; thus they offer primary gain.

Schizophrenic children lack awareness of their own body; their sense of beginnings and endings is impaired, and they are unable to differentiate figure and ground; they are unable to perceive the continuity of objects when the objects are out of sight.

Reduced self-cathexis of libido brings about a diminished sensitivity to pain, observed by Arieti (1955), Goldfarb (1958), Wolman (1966), and others. Some schizophrenic children are unable to localize pain in their own bodies; some of them mutilate themselves because of self-directed aggression or a diffusion of boundaries between themselves and the outer world.

Intellectual and Academic Performance

The school performance of schizophrenic children varies from very poor, resembling mental deficiency, to superb intellectual achievement. In some cases it is a strange combination of both. Thirteen year old Joe, who cannot figure out simple arithmetic questions, can solve algebraic problems and play chess very well. Twelve year old "dull Rosie," who cannot graduate from the fifth grade, is the best in her class in grammar.

Not all schizophrenics are gifted, but poor scholastic performance of a gifted schizophrenic child can be related to his emotional over-involvement and preoccupations. The child who comes to school after witnessing a violent scene between parents, in which one or both of them blame each other for their unhappiness and use the child as a pawn, cannot do well in school. Schizophrenia in childhood is not a defect caused by a trauma; it is a state of continuous irritation, repeated traumas, and perpetuated destructive processes, activated again and again by parental behavior.

The oscillations in the performance of schizophrenic children are largely dependent upon their daily experiences. Ten year old George witnessed a parental fist fight in the morning; the enraged father hit his nagging wife and stormed out of the apartment. George sat in school absentminded, half stuporous, picking his hair, and unable to answer any questions. Our worker spoke with the boy's parents, and they promised to avoid quarrels in the child's presence. George's behavior became less schizophrenic for a few days; the boy responded to the teacher's questions, read and wrote better, paid partial attention to the teacher's explanations, and behaved in the class in a more appropriate manner.

Measurement of intelligence in schizophrenic children is not always valid nor necessarily reliable. Schizophrenia may develop in any human being brought up in the peculiar schizophrenic environment irrespective of his innate intellectual endowment. For years I worked in a clinic diagnosing children with the help of mental tests and projective techniques and later supervised others in that task (Wolman, 1943, 1948). The level of performance of schizophrenic children depended on their mood and on their rapport with the examiner; thus the results could not be taken as a measure of the child's true intelligence. When a schizophrenic child was in a good mood and had established a good rapport with the examiner, he responded well, and very few diagnostic clues in regard to the disorder were observed. Similar conclusions have been reported by other workers (Des Lauriers and Halpern, 1947; Mehr, 1952; and many others). When the child was depressed or frightened or preoccupied, he answered to most questions, "I don't know" or responded in a not-related *non sequitur* manner. Actually schizophrenics always make sense; their communication may report unconscious processes not related to the question but reflecting the child's past experiences and present fears.

Schacter et al. (1962) compared schizophrenic with mentally retarded children. The schizophrenics did not differ significantly from the mentally retarded on play scores relating to things, while both groups were significantly different from the normal children. The schizophrenic and the retarded children engaged less in transportation play and more in disruptive play.

Some schizophrenic children may seem to be untestable when they become absorbed in some autistic mannerism. A schizophrenic child may glance at a picture card and continue tapping, climbing, or masturbating, or even urinate on the blocks in order to wet them.

Schacter et al. (1962) found that the Functioning I.Q. of mentally retarded children was 53.2 (±17.2), 18.1 points higher than that of schizophrenics, which was 35.1 (±10.9). There was, however, no significant difference in the Potential I.Q. of the two groups: the mean I.Q. of the schizophrenic was 74.0 (±28.3) and of the mentally retarded was 84.2 (±23.2). Apparently *schizophrenic children function far below their potential I.Q.* The intellectual functioning of schizophrenic children is definitely inconsistent and often unpredictable, as found by Goldfarb (1961), Winder (1960), Wolman (1946, 1949, 1966), and others.

Wechsler and Jaros (1965) used the WISC method with 150 male schizophrenic children, seven to 15 years old, in Bellevue Psychiatric Hospital. A control group matched for age and I.Q. was selected at random from a population sample used in the original WISC. The schizophrenic children displayed much greater variability than the control group on practically all test items.

Soble (1955) found that thought processes of schizophrenic children also exhibit characteristic disturbances. Schizophrenic children pay attention to tiny details, but they are unable to distinguish the important items from the unimportant ones.

Schizophrenic children are also deviant in their fantasy and play. The exhibit a marked preoccupation with their own fantasy lives, short attention span, and distractiveness.

Many schizophrenic children show speech disturbances. Deviant speech patterns such as muteness, repetitiveness, echolalia, and improper use of personal pronouns reflect their confusion in interpersonal relationships and an inability to perceive boundaries of themselves. Speech defects in schizophrenic children were observed by Goldfarb et al. (1956), such as disturbances in phonation, rhythm, intonation, articulation, volume, and pitch.

Schizophrenic children frequently display peculiar cognitive functions and astonishing memory. In this respect, they resemble adult schizophrenics. A paranoid schizophrenic may recall grievances dating decades back and hold grudges for a great many years. Mahler and Elkisch (1953) related this peculiar talent for retention and recall of the failure of repression.

It seems, however, that this excess memory is related to the schizophrenic hypercathexis. Normally cathexes last much longer than conditioning. The process of extinction makes one forget what has been acquired by conditioning, and the learned connections gradually wear off. Cathexes do not tend to disappear with the lapse of time, and infantile emotional attachment may persist forever. Once emotional energy is cathected in a color, tune, number, a certain type of sexual attraction, etc., it may stay in an individual all his life as his "favorite" color, tune, number, and his "type" of sexually attractive persons. Apparently, cathexes involve more powerful loads of mental energy than conditioning (cf. Wolman, 1966).

The usual process of learning is a process of conditioning, and depends on the initial motivation and consecutive reinforcements. Sometimes certain aspects of education may become reinforced to such an extent as to become one's main occupation and the core of his future life pattern. A schizophrenic child's learning patterns are set early and coincidentally, usually in a wholly irrational way. A schizophrenic cathects certain objects too early and too intensely, to the exclusion of other objects. Father's casual talk about car mechanics may provide a moment of peace and friendly atmosphere and thus steer the child's interest in that direction. A 10 year old boy showed unusual knowledge and understanding of automotive mechanics and a simultaneous lack of understanding for any of the simple problems of science discussed in his class. It was not a lack of intellectual abilities that made him fail in school, but rather the investment of his mental resources in one peculiar and narrow area of interest that became his refuge. In this narrow area, the boy showed unusual memory.

Another possible reason for the excellent memory of schizophrenics is their easy access to the unconscious. Most life experiences register on the preconscious level and are easily accessible, while other experiences register on the unconscious level and are inaccessible or, empirically speaking, forgotten. Schizophrenics may recall minute details from their earliest years that are usually forgotten by normal individuals either by repression or by extinction.

Underachieving

Intellectually gifted children usually perform well in practically all academic subjects, though they may be particularly strong in one subject or a group of subjects. A gifted schizophrenic child may develop mental blocks in several areas. If his father has boasted of his reading or insisted on quick reading to show off to visitors, the child may be afraid to fail his father and refuse to read. To be successful in a schizogenic family is tantamount to being exposed to renewed parental demands and the only way to avoid it is to "fail safe." Many schizophrenic children are *intentional* underchievers, simply to avoid the overdemanding parental pressure. A 12 year old girl who was a borderline schizophrenic told me that she has avoided A marks even in easy subjects, because when she brings home one A mark mother criticizes her for not getting all A marks all the time. It is much easier to avoid mother's criticism by keeping her marks not too high and not too low. She felt that she could not be blamed as long as she did not try too hard; she believed that trying and failing could be catastrophic.

The learning situation represents a great challenge to the schizophrenic child. Learning always involves trials and errors, and the schizophrenic child is afraid of both. His self-esteem is already very low, and his daydreams about great achievements increase the gulf between his desire to be strong and his reality of being weak. When this gulf is painful, he regresses to the infantile hallucinations of omnipotency. Schizophrenic hallucinations always reflect the desire to be the superparent who can create and destroy at will (Wolman, 1966).

Classroom Behavior

Most schizophrenic children would like to be the best in class, but they are afraid to succeed and afraid to fail. The schizophrenic child does not raise his hand to answer the teacher's question because he is not 100 per cent sure that he knows the correct answer. Even when he is sure of the answer, he still cannot be sure that the teacher will call on him, and even if she would she might not like him to give this answer, and if he gave the right answer, wouldn't she demand even a better answer or wouldn't she expect him to always give the right answer? The schizophrenic child feels that the safest thing to do is to keep quiet and withdraw. Schizophrenic children tend to say nothing, do nothing, and feel nothing. They hide behind the evasive answer, "I don't know," even when they know very well. Withdrawal protects one against more demands, against embarrassing situations, and against further loss of the sparce libido energy. *Withdrawal is an energy-saving device,* a sort of economy measure utilized by a child who fears to become involved and forced to give up all his energies in a wasteful object hypercathexis. *Withdrawal is also a protection against being hurt* and against being blamed as the child has been all his years.

School life creates many problems for the schizophrenic child. Pseudo-amentive and autistic children cannot attend a regular school, but less severe schizophrenics can be excellent elementary and high school students, if their intelligence is above average.

I believe that the majority of schizophrenic children should and can attend a regular school and make satisfactory scholastic progress. Their problems lie in the realm of interindividual relations with teachers and children rather than in academic achievement.

Schizophrenic children relate better to adults than to children; they seem to hope that adults will be more understanding, act in a protective, parental manner, and perhaps be less demanding than their own parents are. A schizophrenic child easily forms an attachment to the teacher. If the teacher responds, the child learns eagerly and may even accept the school, gain self-confidence, and relate better to his peers.

Unfortunately, our culture seems to favor the outgoing, expressive, talkative, extrovert type. Many a teacher frowns at the shy, withdrawn child who does not volunteer participation. The shy child craves attention and is afraid of attracting it, but most often the teachers fail to understand him. Many teachers are cold and insecure persons who do not care for the children. Even when the teacher is a good-natured and friendly individual, the chances are that she will not pay attention to the shy and withdrawn little child. Teachers, like most humans, are drawn to the happy, joyous, self-assured children who do not need much attention.

Once again the schizophrenic child has received a harsh lesson. All the teacher wanted was his participation, activity, cooperation, and achievement. The little schizophrenic knows too well that he cannot compete with other children. He has never won over his competing father, and never paid up his debt to his demanding mother. And now, in school, he has failed again.

Even kind and understanding teachers may have difficulties with such a child. A schizophrenic child demands attention and is jealous of the attention shown to other children. When he becomes attached to a teacher, he fears that the teacher may die. Some teachers are insensitive and fail to notice the child's attachment. Some teachers notice and find it burdensome, while others reject the child who demands too much attention.

A schizophrenic child reacts to rejection either by withdrawal or hostility. His reaction depends on his past experiences, but the pattern of reaction is also influenced by the teacher's attitude. When the child feels "left out," he may accept the situation and withdraw even more into fantasy life, daydreaming, and brooding. He may give up all scholastic efforts and regress intellectually. His thought processes, which have improved at the beginning of latency period, may face a setback. As with all other schizophrenics, rejection activates the process of a downward adjustment.

Some teachers do not leave the child alone, but criticize, ridicule, and attack him. The schizophrenic child is an ideal scapegoat. He is often disorganized, not responsive, poorly integrated, passive, afraid to volunteer, seclusive, and inattentive. His books and notebooks are either not kept clean, or he is afraid to open them because they may get dirty. The teacher may voice a sarcastic remark about the child's handwriting, orderliness, or spelling. The teacher's sarcasm may put the entire class into an outburst of laughter, for children, no less than other human beings, have a great deal of cruelty, and they like to achieve a feeling of power by humiliating others. The schizophrenic child may further withdraw, and answer the simplest questions with an evasive and self-protective, "I don't know." An aggressive teacher may use the withdrawn and shy child as an example, and as an opportunity for a display of his or her pedagogic mastery, and ridicule the child more and more. It is quite easy to display one's power at the expense of a lonely, frightened child.

Sometimes the child's reaction is rebellion and active resistance. Hostility elicits hostility and the hurt child may take to arms, hate the teacher, defy her, become destructive and hostile to the school and the children. I have worked with a 10 year old boy who dreamed about stabbing all "teacher's pets" and cutting their bodies into pieces. He also planned to cut out the teacher's tongue so that "she would not say nasty things about kids." Occasionally, he acted out his impulses and hit children, with a heavy stick, on their heads. He also tried to set fire to the school building. His thinking was quite confused; he often mumbled to himself about wars, blood, killings, and death.

The schizophrenic child is afraid of other children. He is afraid because he feels that he is different and has no one to protect him. He is afraid they will attack him and believes that they are his enemies and laugh at him. Hate and fear are inseparable and indispensable ingredients of paranoid schizophrenia (cf. Wolman, 1966, 1970a).

Even when other children are friendly, schizophrenic child may not be able to accept their friendship. Schizophrenic children are often suspicious and afraid of being used and manipulated. Their fear and suspicions may turn into projection of their own hate and develop into ideas of reference.

Most schizophrenic children are so overinvolved with their parents and preoccupied with their family situation that little libido has been left for normal relations with other children. Many schizophrenic children are preoccupied and overinvolved with the problems of their parents to such an extent that they cannot detach themselves and develop sufficient interest for other children.

Yet childhood is childhood even in schizophrenia, and children talk, play, and work together. A schizophrenic child may wish to be the leader or as one 10 year old boy put it, "the big boss." However, the shy, withdrawn, tense schizophrenic does not have a very good chance of becoming a leader. If he is capable of developing friendships, it is usually when he is the follower. The discrepancy between dream and reality increases the tendency to withdraw further into the world of imagined omnipotence and hallucinated power.

Unfortunately, the schizophrenic child hypercathects his little friendships and makes excessive demands on his friends. He is, as a rule, exceedingly jealous and irrational in his demands. Thus, despite his profound desire to have friends, he soon finds himself isolated, rejected, sneered at, and humiliated. Even a well-adjusted child would feel terribly hurt under these circumstances, as children of a persecuted minority group often feel; to a schizophrenic child persecution may become disastrous.

Home Environment

The symptoms of childhood schizophrenia are plastic, changeable, and fluctuating. These fluctuations are caused mainly by interaction with the environment and especially with the child's parents. Schizophrenic behavioral patterns in childhood are less stable than the most unstable behavioral patterns of adult schizophrenics.

Consider 10 year old Peter. While working with the boy, I interviewed both of his parents several times. The father was an exceedingly selfish individual who thought highly of himself and looked down at his wife. His wife felt the same way about her husband. They hated one another intensely, yet they "sacrificed their personal happiness for the child's sake." The mother was overprotective, dictatorial, and symbiotic with the boy to the exclusion of the boy's father. The parents spoke to each other about the boy in his presence; they criticized one another and blamed on each other the boy's shortcomings, as if he were not present or as if he did not understand what they were talking about. The mother told the boy on several occasions that she had not divorced his father only because "the boy needed a father, no matter how bad the father was," but that now the boy was "killing" her.

Occasionally the parents, torn by a feeling of guilt, made a genuine effort to help the boy by being kind to him, but most often the tense interaction between the parents themselves or with the child was fraught with hostile feelings and was therefore devastating to the boy's personality. Occasionally the interparental cold war turned hot and led to verbal or physical clashes between the parents. Each act of violence forced Peter to worry more about his parents, become more fearful and withdrawn, and ultimately aggravated his psychosis.

Similar findings have been reported by other workers (cf. Boatman and Szurek, 1960, pp. 414-416).

Those children who are mute or who talk about themselves in the third person are often children whose parents talk about them in their presence as if they were not there. . . . It is frequent for a parent to answer for a child when the child is spoken to. . . . Many parents behave toward the child as if he were stupid. . . . Threats about her [mother's] wish never to return again may also appear, only to be followed by renewed efforts to get the child to say he loves her. . . . Some parents urge a child to dress or feed himself, to take over once he starts, presumably because he is so slow or clumsy. . . . Lack of discussion between parents is very frequent. . . . Angry projections, even if unverbalized, are frequent between the parents and toward the child. . . .Each parent has experienced intensified unconscious needs for exclusive, all-loving, undemanding, tender care and understanding from the spouse.

Some mothers treat the child as if he were an inanimate object and their sole property. As a result, many psychotic children do not have a conception of personal property. They take things which do not belong to them, and they give away their things. Possession is a concept that is gradually acquired; it starts with the anal stage, and the anal stage is of special importance in the formation of schizophrenia. Schizogenic mothers are usually very demanding in toilet training; many of them use enemas, and later they take away the toys they have given to the child as if they belonged to the mother and not to the child.

Mary was 12. She was a "bad girl," according to her mother. She was, however, a good infant, obedient, early toilet trained, and neat. Now Mary is described by her mother as stubborn and rebellious and one who breaks things and screams. Mary does not want to study and is afraid of people. She has no property of her own, for her mother has everything under her control. The mother exercised strict control over Mary's bowel movements, regulated her meals, and forced the food in and feces out. The mother never allowed Mary to play in the sandbox in the park with the other children because the sand was dirty and the other children were not neatly dressed. Besides, the mother explained, children carry germs. Now the 12 year old is afraid of children, germs, and mud.

The mother has controlled Mary's toys, crayons, paper cutouts, dolls, songs, words, and thoughts. She took Mary's toys out of the closet, and when she decided that Mary had had enough playing, she put them back. The mother played with Mary whenever *she* was in the mood to and forbade Mary to play with the "dirty, bad" children on the street. Now Mary fears bad children and bad people, and most of all she fears her own thoughts of death. What will happen when mother dies? Is she, Mary, killing her, as her mother says frequently?

The mother dressed and undressed Mary, washed and scrubbed her daily. Mother's symbiotic needs have been satisfied by handling the girl as if she were a piece of property, sort of an inanimate object.

Now Mary does not know what belongs to whom. She takes things that belong to other children, and she gives away her toys. She cannot concentrate in school. When the teacher talks, Mary doodles, daydreams, or makes strange grimaces. She envies other children; they can talk, sing, and play. One little girl tried to be friendly with Mary. Since the girl lived in the next house, she came over (her mother allowed her out of the house) to play with Mary. But although Mary's mother had constantly nagged, "Why don't you make friends?" she did not like Mary's friend because of her religion. And so Mary lost her only friend and was growing more lonely, more fearful, and more confused. The world seemed to be cold and hostile, and most of all Mary feared that she herself was a "bad girl."

Acting Out

A schizophrenic child of average intelligence knows well what is right and wrong and fears to do wrong, but most often his ego fails in the exercise of self-control. Usually the child knows when he does something wrong and in his inner desperate struggle against his impulses, he approaches the catatonic type. Sometimes he does not care what he does and acts in a "I don't care" manner, soiling himself, breaking things, and laughing at the sight of the damage. Obviously such behavior comes close to the hebephrenic type in adult schizophrenia.

When the ego defenses fail, the schizophrenic child is most likely to act out his confused sexual impulses. Schizophrenics, as a result of the peculiar confusion of sex and age roles in their family, are frequently confused in regard to their own sex identification. Schizophrenic children do not have much opportunity for development of rational inhibitions and sublimations. Frequently, they act in an uninhibited, polymorphously perverted manner. Geleerd (1949) described a case of a 7½ year old boy who was "highly excitable and having outstanding anal and sexual habits. He was supposed to have grabbed the penises of other boys . . . or he would chase the other children excitedly with feces on a stick" (p. 311).

I remember an 11 year old boy who insisted that the nurse or attendant wipe his behind after elimination. Then he would grab the nurse's finger and push it into his anus, and rub his back against the nurse's body with obvious signs of sexual arousal. A 10 year old schizophrenic girl seduced little boys, having regular sex intercourse with them; she also indulged in homosexual play with girls and was frequently seen masturbating in public. Some of these children partly repress and partly displace their sexual impulses; in such cases, their sexual acting out takes on the bizarre patterns of touching objects in a fetishistic manner, such as playing with water pipes, digging holes, collecting sticks, looking under sinks, etc.

Acting out of destructive impulses takes on several forms in childhood schizophrenia. When a schizophrenic child, not being in a tantrum, acts negativistically, defying his parents and destroying objects, he is usually testing them. He tests and waits to see what is going to happen. In contradistinction to a psychopathic child who always believes that he is right, a schizophrenic child knows that he is "bad" and does wrong things. A psychopath invents excuses and pleads innocent, for he believes that he is entitled to grab, hurt, defy, and exploit others (see Wolman, 1970a).

A schizophrenic knows well that he is wrong. He tries to control himself and, as a rule, fails. Then he feels depressed and guilty. Sometimes he tests his parents; will they reject him, if he is not compliant? How can he be sure that they love him? Do they love him only when he is a perfect child and hate him as soon as he fails?

When hostility turns inward, the schizophrenic child mutilates himself by pulling his hair, scratching his face, and banging his head. Quite often he provokes fights in order to be beaten up and to prove to himself that he is bad and that the world is hostile and retaliatory. When the inner pressures become unbearable, the schizophrenic child projects his own hostility in a paranoid fashion, believing that the world has ganged up against him.

Sometimes he tests his own destructive impulses. Is he really a dangerous person? Is he really the cause of his parents' sicknesses and misfortunes? Is he as bad as his mother keeps telling him? Does he really make his mother sick, and will she soon die because of him? This is an unbearable thought—it makes him feel weird, but this is what his mother keeps repeating.

Bettelheim (1955, p. 253) gives an interesting description of a schizophrenic girl: "When Mary discovered that her destructive wishes and violent attacks did not damage us [and] the other children . . . she began doubting whether she was as destructive as she feared, and hence whether she was actually the cause of her mother's death."

Sometimes a schizophrenic's acting out is no longer testing, for a slight provocation may throw the child into a state of uncontrollable aggressiveness. Also Boatman and Szurek (1960, p. 399) noticed the vicious self-assaultiveness in schizophrenic children, such as head banging, face slapping, tongue biting, face scratching, etc. When interfered with, self-aggressive behavior may turn against others. I have seen this phenomenon and its reversals ever so often: an assault on others, when interfered with by an adult, led to a vicious attack on oneself; and interrupted assault on oneself turned into an assault on the interfering nurse.

In manifest adult schizophrenics unconscious flooded conscious. Hence delusions, hallucinations, irrational ways of thinking, wayward association, condensations, and pictorial symbolic expressions bear witness to the influx of primary processes. In childhood schizophrenics there is more fluidity in the transition from secondary to primary processes. A schizophrenic child does not live in a world of fantasy all the time. For instance:

Little Steve knows that he is being tested. He knows that his mother calls the man who talks to her "Doctor." He is aware of all that, yet he is not sure what all this is about. For a while he responds to me, then something distracts his attention. He stares blankly into space, and does not react to my questions, as if I were not there any more. Then he gets a frightened look in his eyes and answers in an unrelated way. After a while he begins to ask me questions about people being dead. He does not wait for my answer; he as'ːs me, "Is he really a bad boy and that's why his mother is sick?" "Yes", he answers himself, "he knows that Steve is a very bad boy." Then his thoughts jump to another topic, seemingly not related: "Must all people die?"

Fear of Death

Normal children may experience fears and have a rich fantasy life. However, they are usually able to distinguish between true and "pretended" experience. Well-adjusted children know that they "make up stories." A schizophrenic child is not sure any longer; he easily loses the distinction between truth and story especially when he is upset, in fear or rage. In emotional upheavals schizophrenic children are out of contact with reality.

All children have fears, but the more protection they receive from their parents, the easier it is for them to overcome their fears. A schizophrenic child is a child who does not feel protected. *Fear of death* is the outstanding feature of all hypervectorial disorders, both in childhood and adulthood. The manifestly psychotic child is not only preoccupied with this fear, but most frequently identifies himself with the killers or with the killed. A nine year old boy, described by Despert (1955, pp. 248-249) "created a world of his own where destructive, frightening, horrible things are going on all the time. Most of his utterances were incoherent." Most of his play was acting out the theme of killing and being killed. Another child had garbled speech, infantile behavior, showed extreme hostility in her fantasies of violent death that involved her parents and siblings. World destruction fantasies frequently ended with a statement: "Everything is destroyed except me—I'm too smart—I'm a God" (*ibid.,* p. 250). The schizophrenic drive for power borders in this case on delusion of omnipotence.

The fear of death in schizophrenic children is experienced as a panic of ceasing to be oneself. The feeling of *not-me,* of not being oneself represents a loss of identity and a sign of decline of the ego. The schizophrenic child often experiences these panic-producing feelings. Depersonalization and the feeling of not being oneself are signs of the oncoming breakdown in latent schizophrenics (Bychowski, 1952; Federn, 1952; Wolman, 1957, 1966). Some children never experience a clear-cut feeling of being themselves; the *not-me* feeling is experienced frequently.

Some workers (R. D. Rabinowitch and S. Dubo, quoted by W. J. Hendrickson, 1952) see in the loss of identity the

core problem, pathognomic to the illness. . . . The child's inability to experience as a clear-cut self-percept and to appreciate identities, their boundaries and limits. . . . It is as though the child merged diffusely with objects in his environment. The term 'dysidentity' would seem to accurately describe this basic problem. . . . An earlier traditional view of the major symptomatology of childhood schizophrenia as being a social withdrawal and an exorbitant fantasy life, with perhaps delusions and hallucinations, has proved invalid and has clouded the basic issues. In many cases, and especially early in the course of the disease, these symptoms may not be present at all. The problem of dysidentity is basic, however. . . .

Fear of death, as in other types of hypervectorial disorders, forces more regression and more downward adjustment.

Physical Symptoms

Schizophrenic children display a variety of physical symptoms and physical diseases. Vasovegetative dysfunctioning is apparent in excessive liability or lack of responsiveness in vasomotor behavior. Schizophrenic children are prone to be flushed and perspire profusely. Many schizophrenic children are exceedingly pale, oversensitive to cold weather, and have cold, blue extremities. Their reaction to the usual physical diseases of childhood is unpredictable and disproportionate to the severity of the illness. Schizophrenic children sometimes develop severe infections with temperatures that are not high or show high temperatures with minor colds and infections.

The physiological functions of daily life are often highly disturbed. Eating, sleeping, and elimination patterns are irregular, imposing undue hardship on their mothers, who complain about the infant's disorderly conduct being unaware of the fact that the infant merely reacts to his environment.

Motor coordination is often delayed or disturbed in schizophrenic children. Their uneven physical and mental development results in awkwardness, lack of precision, and lack of decisiveness. Sometimes motor independence and skill develop early in childhood and as the schizophrenic process becomes aggravated, a deterioration in motor coordination occurs. Many schizophrenic children fear to walk alone or ride a tricycle. Some of them can never learn swimming or ice skating. The early reflexes tend to persist, and some schizophrenic children perpetuate choreoathetotic activities, retained from the first years of life and developed into a compulsive behavioral pattern. Certain mannerisms also seem to persevere into later childhood, so that it is not uncommon to find a schizophrenic child rocking his head or sucking his fingers.

Postural reflexes also indicate infantile perseveration or regression. The speed and ease with which schizophrenic children adopt any posture placed on them resembles adult catatonia. Bender tested the postural reflex. She had the child stand with arms outstretched in front and his eyes closed, and turned the child's head from side to side. A normal child responds by turning his body in the direction of his head, but a schizophrenic child reacts with whirling motion and continues this motion spontaneously. Rotating, rocking, whirling, and rhythmic repetition motions belong to major motor activity patterns of child schizophrenics, as well as facial grimaces, grinning, and exaggerated postures and actions.

The voice of a schizophrenic child is often wooden-like, lacking modulation, and sometimes with sing-song intonations. According to Bender, "The voice sounds as if it doesn't belong to the person, as if it's not sure of its ego boundaries." The child demonstrates an inability to recognize or care for his bodily secretions. Bender attributes this to the child's inability to locate the periphery of his body. Another interpretation relates this symptom to inadequate cathexis of one's own body, typical of all schizophrenics (Wolman, 1966).

3. LATENT SCHIZOPHRENIA IN CHILDHOOD

Dependence-Independence

Latent schizophrenia develops in children when their superego is strong enough to prevent the victory of the id over the ego. The ego, while subservient to the superego, is still capable of testing reality and exercise a tenuous control, but it is unable to prevent occasional outbursts of vehement emotion. The child's daily behavior resembles a volcano that has not yet erupted; it is the quiet before the storm.

Many actions of the latent schizophrenic child are dictated not by practical but by moralistic considerations. Normally a child refrains from getting himself into trouble because he fears he may hurt himself; the reality principle overrules the pleasure principle. In latent schizophrenic children it is the superego and not the ego that imposes self-restraint, for the fear of hurting mother looms larger than the fear of hurting himself.

The latent schizophrenic child is preoccupied with the fear of his own death, of that his parents and his friends. The only way he can ward off the fear of death is by adhering to rigid and inflexible rules. The latent schizophrenic child is more compulsive than the adult obsessive-compulsive neurotic. To be orderly, punctilious, neat, and clean is a matter of life or death for the child.

Although the latent schizophrenic is more compulsive than the obsessional neurotic, he is less successful in his repressions, displacements, and reaction formations. As long as his ego exercises partial control, his behavior is more rigid than the behavior of the obsessive-compulsive neurotic, but his ego easily and frequently loses its grip over the unconscious impulses and his behavior occasionally turns psychotic.

One of the outstanding features of latent schizophrenia in childhood is the fluctuation between the neurotic ego protective and psychotic ego deficiency symptoms (Ekstein and Wallerstein, 1954; Wolman, 1957, 1966); the overt behavior varies from normal to bizarre. Some latent schizophrenics display compulsive gestures, tics, and grinning; some talk to themselves, eat in a messy way, are dirty and disorganized; some others, and sometimes the same children in a different mood, are exceedingly neat, overconscientious in their work, and self-controlled. The same child can be sloppy and pedantic, helpless and ingenious, fearful and fearless (Brask, 1959).

The latent schizophrenic child is a child who has been forced to be a model child. He was not allowed to fight back when hurt by his parents; whenever he rebelled against them, he was made to feel that he was killing his weak parents and, therefore, would be lonely and doomed to death. He was constantly blamed for defending himself and for not being an angel-like, subservient, and always obedient child.

Thus he develops inner defense mechanisms to prevent his allegedly evil nature from coming through. These are his neurotic ego protective defenses that, in a way, delay the onset of manifest psychosis.

Sometimes the child makes a strange compromise between his angel-like intentions and devil-like impulses. He becomes a "hostile angel" or a "loving devil," who loves one thing and finds in his great love justification for his hate and cruelty toward anyone else. Such an extreme rationalization is typical for character neurosis (Wolman, 1966, 1970a).

Sometimes a desperate struggle goes on between the hostile impulses and the controlling apparatus. This desperate struggle characterizes latent schizophrenia.

Latent schizophrenic children are torn by the *dependence-independence* conflict. To grow up means to be independent, but to be independent means to rely on one's own judgment, to care less for mother, and to abandon her. Thus, growth creates guilt feelings and "dependence-independence" becomes a major conflict. To stay where one is and to avoid growth may seem to be the choice method which reflects the schizophrenic, morbid regressive adjustment.

Not all children succumb to their parasitic-symbiotic mothers and parasitic fathers and accept overdependence on them. Some children fantasize and wish mother and/or father dead; then they could be free and subject no more to slavery and the self-destructive object hypercathexis. The conflict between dependence and independence aggravates and becomes a conflict between being good and weak or strong and hostile. The child wants to be strong, but at the same time he fears to be left alone, unsupported and exposed to mortal dangers. Some children "solve" this problem by being overly passive, overdependent, compliant in their waking life, and active and aggressive in their dreams and daydreams. With their shaky personality structure, the hostile wishes and dreams may turn into reality at slight provocation.

Some of these children have been described by Geleerd (1960, p. 158) as "borderline states." These children show lack of tolerance to frustration, emotional immaturity, unevenness of development, uncontrollable id impulses, lack of social adaptation, plus a variety of neurotic symptoms.

They were in contact with reality and not delusional. But when they were alone or when they felt frustrated, they very easily withdrew into fantasy life or had severe temper outbursts. . . . Like the much younger child, they could not function in a group since this meant sharing the love object.

Classroom Behavior

Latent schizophrenic children can be as good students as their intellectual abilities permit, provided that they feel secure and accepted. An unfriendly teacher or rejecting classmates may cause them to fail in all subjects and even refuse to attend classes. However, many latent schizophrenic children are diligent students and do well in school.

Classmates represent a difficult challenge. The latent schizophrenic child easily becomes overinvolved with another child and, inevitably, hurt by unwillingness or inability of the other child to respond in the same way.

Eleven year old Terry developed a profound attachment to the most popular girl in the class. Terry helped her girl friend and served her in many ways in schoolwork, bringing snacks and candies, etc. Terry was not buying her friend's friendship; she was genuinely attached and loyally faithful. When her girl friend was ungrateful or disloyal, Terry sobbed through sleepless nights.

The latent schizophrenic child has little if any chance to be popular with the crowd. Children in the latency period are often clannish, form cliques, and become hostile to those who "do not belong." Manifest schizophrenics, with their bizarre behavior, invite persecution; latent schizophrenics, with their bashful, awkward behavior, invite ostracism or at least a flat rejection or a cold shoulder.

The rejected child may withdraw even more or become aggressive or both. Most latent schizophrenic children blame themselves. Their superego exercises dictatorial power, and they are prone to blame themselves for whatever injustice is done to them. A 12 year old girl felt that her mother was right to enforce her to take care of her younger sister; her teacher was right in not paying attention to her and favoring the bright, good-looking, and smiling girls.

This hostility, turned inward, may sometimes return to the outer world; latent schizophrenic children may provoke aggression from their schoolmates by teasing, calling names, taking things away, and even pushing and hitting. A manic depressive is a coward; a psychopath is aggressive but only attacks easy targets and avoids being beaten; a schizophrenic is often "overcourageous" and attacks without self-protection. He may attack bigger children and invite defeat and humiliation as if to prove that he deserves the punishment he receives. At the same time, his provocation to fight enables him to discharge part of the accumulated destrudo energy.

Paranoid ideas are frequent in a latent-schizophrenic child. If these ideas prevail and he begins to see himself surrounded by enemies, his mental status is a manifest and not latent psychosis any longer. Latent schizophrenic children (Geleerd, 1946, p. 272)

display a far lesser degree of control over their aggressive actions than do other children of the same age. Also they show a lack of control over their anal and sexual impulses. . . . In most of their activities they tend to present an uncontrollably impulsive behavior. . . . Their temper tantrums differ from those of the normal or neurotic child and their aggressiveness is dangerous both to themselves and to the environment. The child is out of control with reality and believes himself to be persecuted . . . [and] becomes more paranoid when treated with firmness. He considers it proof of his paranoid ideas. . . . The tantrums increase in violence with the age of the child.

Similar observations were reported by Ekstein and Wallerstein (1954) on several borderline cases of childhood schizophrenia. Under the mildest stress their ego defenses fall apart and the child plunges into world-destructive or even oral-canabilistic fantasies.

Sometimes these children burst out into laughter when they act destructively, as if experiencing a triumph and a great feeling of power. Some latent schizophrenic children like to crack jokes, tease, and make practical jokes. These childish pranks serve a definite purpose of increasing their self-esteem. The mechanism used is the use of destructive power. In adult schizophrenics the drive for power frequently takes on the form of delusions and hallucinations. The omnipotence fantasies of schizophrenic children come close to the pattern of delusion.

Home Environment

Parents are frequently the targets of the child's outbursts of destrudo. An eleven year old girl attacked her father, hit and scratched him, and used abusive language whenever she had any difficulty with her despotic mother, as if she were saying: "Why do you neglect me and never offer the expected protection!"

The more the parents quarrel between themselves, the more they stimulate the child's destrudo. In latent schizophrenia the inner struggle between object-directed and self-directed destrudo is quite pronounced. The child is afraid he may do wrong and that he will be blamed. This fear of one's own destructiveness creates the compulsive need for keeping everything under control, namely, himself, the parents, the household, the neighborhood, etc. On many occasions I have seen parents bowing to the whims of a latent schizophrenic child in complete surrender to the child's irrational wishes, fears, and temper tantrums. The terrorized parents try to please and bribe the child, being unaware of the fact that their weakness increases his anxiety and provokes more violent outbursts.

The child insists on a strict and rigid routine in daily life and allows no changes. When the mother is not home when the child comes home from school, or when the father is late for supper, when a piece of furniture is moved out of its place, when anything new and unfamiliar happens, the child gets into panic and rage. Moving to a new neighborhood, change of school, the departure or, even worse, the death of a relative or friend are experienced by the child as major catastrophies that may elicit an overtly psychotic behavior. In such an outbreak the child may become blindly aggressive, attacking himself and others without being fully aware of what he is doing. He may also develop catatonic or hebephrenic symptoms.

Latent schizophrenics function with a precarious balance and tenuous ego control. Their ego is weak and desperately struggles to comply with the superego and to control the id. In this constant tension, the ego cannot take much frustration. When a manifest psychotic child is hurt by rejection or failure, he may react with an "I don't care" attitude. A latent schizophrenic views his failure as a major disaster.

Sometimes the fear of failing and being blamed by mother is strongly connected with a fear of excelling and outdistancing father. A 13 year old, very bright boy was keeping his school record on a persistently low average. He was afraid to fail; poor marks invited mother's never-ending accusations. However, whenever he got excellent marks, his mother was full of joy but his father, who had not received formal education and was a laborer, seemed to feel upset and apparently depressed by the success of his son, in whom he saw a competitor for his wife's favor. When the father died, the boy's school marks improved substantially.

4. SCHIZOPHRENIA IN ADOLESCENCE

The Onset

The onset of schizophrenia has frequently been associated with adolescence. Undoubtedly adolescence is a time of great emotional changes and personality formation, and several workers believe that adolescence is a period of a "normal" challenge to one's mental health. Yet even the most stormy adolescence of a normal youngster has little, if anything, in common with a mild schizophrenic in this age.

Schizophrenia does not start at adolescence. Most cases are "overstayed" cases of childhood schizophrenia. Some are cases of childhood schizophrenia that have improved for a while and then, under the impact of biological growth and social role readjustment faced by all adolescents, slowly or rapidly regressed into manifest psychosis (cf. Beres, 1956). There is, however, fairly good reason to believe that adolescence may activate latent conflicts and aggravate the already existing hypervectorial disorder.

The aggravation of symptoms and personality deterioration may be caused by both biological and social factors. The growth of the organism, with its metabolic and endocrine changes, has a disturbing impact on all adolescents and represents a challenge to the shaky personality structure of a hypervectorial neurotic or latent psychotic.

The other challenge comes from the environment. Most parents of adolescent schizophrenics whom I interviewed seem to be utterly disoriented, angry at their children, spouses, and themselves, and acting in a self-contradictory and usually self-defeating manner. In cases where the adolescent has been a quite subdued child for years, neurotic or character neurotic (see the next chapter), and begins to act out at puberty, his parents seem to be shocked and bewildered. They cannot understand the sudden change that has occurred in their "model child," and ascribe the change to the school, the neighbors, or any other outside influence. Most often the parents resort to severe punishment, being unaware of the destructive import of punishment on schizophrenia.

The adolescents with a sudden onset have for years struggled against their hostile impulses, and punishment destroys the last vestiges of self-control. A 14 year old schizophrenic boy who set fire to his house was "taking revenge" for the severe beating he received from his father. A $13\frac{1}{2}$ year old girl practiced unrestrained sexual promiscuity when her parents called her a prostitute. Aretic tendencies, barely repressed in latency, may break through in a full-blown paranoid or catatonic schizophrenia. Parental anger often serves as a catalyst.

At this stage the parental behavior does not cause schizophrenia but rather is reduced to a precipitating role. Even well-wishing and good-natured parents are helpless when confronted with a sudden schizophrenia, whether it turns paranoid, catatonic, or hebephrenic. Simple deterioration symptoms such as gradual withdrawal, depression, and passivity are least spectacular and least noticeable, but they are prognostically the worst ones.

Simple deterioration schizophrenia develops gradually after years of neurotic, character neurotic, or latent psychotic (hypervectorial) disorders. The three other schizophrenic syndromes may also have an insidious onset, after years of gradual deterioration. In such cases most parents are utterly discouraged and resigned. I saw cases where the entire family bowed to the most irrational whims of a latent schizophrenic child. When finally the $14\frac{1}{2}$ year old boy stopped talking and remained in a catatonic stupor, his family took it without much dismay and sent him away to a mental hospital.

Symonds and Herman (1957) studied hospitalized adolescent girls, age 12-18, with intelligence level ranging from defective to bright normal. The authors grouped these girls as follows: (1) The girls in the first group had made adequate adjustments to life and had serious disturbances only with the onset of manifest schizophrenia. These girls were believed to be well until they reached adolescence, when they developed withdrawal symptoms, refused to go out, and avoided people. Most of them refused to go to school, and some of them developed auditory hallucinations. (2) The girls of the second group had serious behavior and personality problems in childhood. They were truants, quarrelsome, and had been caught stealing. They had difficulties in school, and were paranoid and aggressive. (3) The girls of the third group had been maladjusted in their childhood. Their behavior was bizarre, and they were never liked by other children.

Prior to hospitalization, the girls practiced prostitution, extortion, and kidnapping. Some of them attempted suicide and genocide. All girls came from broken homes or homes torn by interparental strife.

The peer relations in adolescence seem to have a serious effect upon schizophrenics. Some preadolescent schizophrenic children had had friends and companions and did not lack the sociability for relating to their peers, but most of them appeared to be isolated.

Many schizophrenics had been considered "good boys" or "model boys" by their demanding parents and were obedient to their mothers. They hesitated, however, to fight or even to participate in rough, body contact sports. Most of them had been ridiculed and discouraged by abuse and rejection and had withdrawn from all social contacts. Most schizophrenic adolescents are lonely and feel that they are "different." The isolation from peers and the feeling of rejection has aggravated their condition (Weinberg, 1960; Wolman, 1966).

Sexual Behavior

Adolescence brings about the recurrence of Oedipus conflicts combined with increased sexual tensions. "There is a necessity as Freud has stated to attain genital primacy over pregenital sexual drives which appears to be an important psychic function," (Neubauer and Steinhert, 1952, p. 130). "This consideration alone indicates that true understanding of psycho-dynamic aspects in relationship to adolescence, leads us back to a history of earlier developmental states." We must first understand the structure of the organism before understanding the process that attacks adolescent life. Neubauer feels that we should not limit our understanding of the psychodynamic aspects of adolescence to a repetition of earlier phases without due consideration of the additional capacities which the person has obtained in reaching adolescence. "Adolescence seems to have at is disposal Oedipal and therefore psychoneurotic conflict constellations. The schizophrenic process shows deviant mechanisms of much earlier life in which a more serious regression or fixation to a pre-Oedipal state of development through external or internal traumata has occurred" (*ibid.*, p. 131). Fusion of the psychoneurotic mannerisms of the Oedipus stage with those of the pre-Oedipal stage are part of the pathology of schizophrenia in the adolescent.

Schizophrenics have difficulties in relating to the opposite sex. These relationships are affected by their confused notion about their own sexual identity, which they have had since childhood. Many preschizophrenics are confused by their parents and have not been able to identify with either of them. Hence most schizophrenics have no sex role models to follow. These conflicts concerning their sexual identity come to a manifest climax during adolescence, when their sex impulses become more imperative and when age mates compel association with the opposite sex. Because of their isolation from their peers they have not acquired the skills and techniques for dating and courtship. They are therefore vulnerable because of their inner conflicts about sex and their ignorance of the appropriate manner in dating. Most female adolescent schizophrenics are unable to cope with interpersonal relation with the opposite sex and seek the protective companionship of older men upon whom they become very dependent. Some schizophrenics solve their conflicts by virtually denying or repressing their sex pursuits or refraining from associations with the opposite sex (Weinberg, 1960).

The sexual behavior of adolescent schizophrenic girls follows a variety of extreme behavioral patterns. Some girls practice indiscriminate promiscuity, while others avoid any sexual contacts at all. Since most of these girls think very little of themselves and do not expect anyone to be interested in them, they avoid any contact that could end in a disappointment.

Seventeen year old Mary Ann maintained that all men want from girls is sex and nothing else. She was highly critical of all men and accused them of chasing after "fresh flesh." She believed that she was physically unattractive and, therefore, that no man would ever pay attention to her as a person.

When a 22 year old man began to call her and expressed profound interest in her, she reacted in a sarcastic and hostile manner to his advances. Apparently, the young man sincerely liked her, but Mary Ann did not believe that anyone ever could like her. Her hostile behavior finally achieved its objectives; the young man stopped calling her and Mary Ann "proved" to herself that no one likes her and no one is trustworthy. When he began to date one of her acquaintances, she went into a deep depression and withdrawal and harbored suicidal thoughts.

This self-defeating behavioral pattern repeats itself in practically all adolescent schizophrenics, whether they abstain from sexual relations or indulge in unrestrained and unselective promiscuity.

Lea was 18 years old when she was referred to me for treatment. She was a bright, good-looking, tall blonde girl with a pleasant smile. She was shy and withdrawn, and cried frequently and was diagnosed as a latent schizophrenic.

Her life history was rather eventful. When she was 10, her father tried to seduce her and indulged for a year or more in quite intense sexual play. When her mother discovered the incestuous relationship, she broke up with her husband, with whom she quarrelled for years.

Two years later the mother remarried. Lea acted seductively toward her stepfather who impressed her by his vigor, aggressiveness, and arrogance. Soon she became his mistress.

When her mother became suspicious, Lea began to avoid her stepfather. The frustrated man became vindicative and jealous and did not allow his 15 year old stepdaughter to go out with boys. Under disguise of parental authority and high moralistic principles, the stepfather punished Lea severely for coming late, failing in school, and any other transgressions. When he saw her talking on the street with a boy schoolmate, he beat her mercilessly.

Lea somehow arrived at the conclusion that she was being rejected by her stepfather because she refused to have sexual relations with him. Sex was apparently the only thing she had to offer, for she herself as a person did not deserve any attention or friendship.

Pretty soon Lea became "popular" with the boys. She slept with whoever "was nice to her" and she began to believe that now the boys liked her. She was raped on several occasions and had two abortions. When she first came to my office, she was firmly convinced that no man could ever be interested in her unless she went to bed with him, and she contemplated becoming a call girl.

Schizophrenics, as such, do not have particularly strong or particularly weak sexual impulses, and there is nothing specifically schizophrenic in their sexual desires and preferences. Two elements in sexual behavior are, however, typically schizophrenic, namely, the disbalance in *self-regulation* and confusion as to one's *psychosexual role*.

The first applies to the above-described cases and to the cases described by Symonds and Herman (1957). Some schizophrenic adolescents overdo in self-restraint and avoid any contact with people of the opposite sex, though most of them have lost all self-control and indulge in limitless promiscuity. Many schizophrenic adolescents, males and females, find in sexual activity the only way to "prove" their own value and use sex as an escape from a devastating inferiority feeling and doubts concerning their proper gender.

The doubts of adolescent schizophrenics concerning their psychosexual roles are rooted in their intrafamilial experiences. Normal parents do not involve their children in their personal problems. Whether their family life is or is not gratifying, they avoid informing children of interparental relationships and problems.

Schizophrenic parents notoriously implicate their children in their personal life. Being disappointed in each other and emotionally frustrated, they expect from the child (who will become schizophrenic) all the affection and love they have expected in vain from their spouses. Thus, when the child reaches puberty and is naturally inclined to experience strong sexual arousal, he acts as if he or she were an adult lover, lacking all sexual restraint. Children who have had sexual experience with their parents either continue unrestrained sexual practices or, by reaction formation, develop strong anti-sexual aversions.

In many instances, frustrated parents seduce the child of the same sex. Such an emotional and sometimes physical seduction increases the child's confusion. Sixteen year old Debora felt that she was the sole moral support and lover of her poor mother and tried to fill the vacuum in her mother's life by assuming father's role. When she was sent away to a boarding school, she developed a passionate sexual attachment to the housemother and later became actively homosexual in regard to her roommate.

A similar process takes place in male schizophrenics.

Take 17 year old Joe, whose schizogenic family prevented the establishment of a proper sex-age role. As a little boy he was not a little boy who will eventually grow up and become a big man. Early in childhood he became his mother's confessor and accomplice. His negative Oedipal involvement with his father was stimulated by both parents, and he was put into a competitive position with his mother. His sentimental and affectionate father sought solace in Joe's love for him; hugging, kissing, and even sleeping together well into adolescence were not unusual occurrences. When he first came to my office, he displayed coy, girlish mannerisms, and told me what brands of eau de cologne he and his mother "adore." He was afraid of boys and avoided sports that required physical contact. He was not actively homosexual, but he has spent all his time with his mother and sister and blamed his two uncles and soon also myself for homosexual advances toward him.

Aggressive and Self-Destructive Behavior

Most schizophrenics struggle against their own pent-up hostility, which they could not vent in childhood. In paranoid schizophrenia this hostility is projected onto others and thus one's own behavior is rationalized; in catatonic schizophrenia the efforts of self-control lead to mutism, stupor, etc., with occasional violent acting out; in hebephrenic schizophrenia the defenses collapse and patients act out uninhibited hostility; in simple deterioration cases the hostility turns inward.

Adolescent schizophrenics display all the above-mentioned types of aggressive and self-destructive behavior. Some of them, especially in the latent psychotic stage, cautiously avoid violence and fear clashes. Some others become exceedingly aggressive as if perpetuating the *aretic* syndrome of childhood schizophrenia with distinct paranoid features.

In most of these late aretic cases, aggression dominates the picture while other symptoms are cast aside or diminish. The aretic adolescent becomes quarrelsome and provocative as if looking for excuses to start a fight.

Lauretta Bender maintains that many adolescent schizophrenics show a marked physiological, intellectual, emotional, and social improvement (Bender, 1956), while becoming juvenile delinquents. A follow-up of schizophrenic children whose schizophrenic symptoms diminished at puberty found their behavior similar to that of a psychopath (Tec, 1955). Bender and her associates noticed antisocial behavior, antagonistic to authorities, aggressive and sexually impulsive. Occasional delusions were channelled in terms of a negativistic or a paranoid philosophy. Adolescent delinquent schizophrenics usually justify their antisocial behavior in a self-righteous manner. Bender called these adolescents, *schizoid psychopathic* or *pseudo-psychopathic* (Bender, 1956).

As mentioned before, there is a distinct difference between schizophrenic and psychopathic aggressiveness. Psychopaths fight for gain; they steal, loot, rape, and murder for money, sex, victory, and feeling of power.

Schizophrenics become aggressive either when they believe themselves to be under attack (in paranoid schizophrenia) or when they flare up in a senseless fury and anger with no rational reason, for their actions are of no advantage to themselves (in catatonic and hebephrenia). Adolescent schizophrenics often commit outrageous crimes against people and property with no gain or purpose. Quite often they provoke strong adversaries, probably with an unconscious desire to be hurt and punished.

Suicide

Many adolescent schizophrenics, tormented by a feeling of guilt for their thought of, but not implemented, hostile acts against their parents and the entire world, turn their aretic impulses inward and attack themselves. Self-defeating and self-destructive attitudes are quite common among adolescent schizophrenics. Suicide is the culmination of self-directed destructiveness.

Most often suicidal attempts indicate the onset of the simple deterioration syndrome of manifest schizophrenia. A latent schizophrenic who was a "model child" may not be able to cope any longer with his deep feeling of guilt and depression, and may decide that he does not deserve to live. He evaluates himself and his entire past as a continuous chain of failures. He grows apathetic and gradually withdraws from all social contacts. Afraid of his own sexual and aggressive impulses and giving up all hope, he may decide to put an end to his misery.

Males outnumber females in each group of successful suicides, but females outnumber males in attempted suicides by an equally large number. Toolan (1962) hypothesizes that boys find it easier to be aggressive towards themselves than do girls. Suicide is the second ranking cause of death among university students.

Toolan found that of 900 admissions to the children's and adolescent services of Bellevue Hospital 102 were for suicidal attempts and threats. There was a steady increase from the age of eight; 18 were under 12 years of age, and 84 out of 102 were in the 12 to 17 age group. The vast majority of the suicide cases were diagnosed as schizophrenic.

None of my patients has ever committed suicide, but I have treated several schizophenics who had attempted suicide in their teens and a great many who had harbored suicidal thoughts at that time.

Other Symptoms

Schizophrenia in adolescence offers a variety of behavioral patterns, and its symptomatology is exasperatingly diversified. Some adolescents remain prepsychotic; some display pseudo-amentive, symbiotic, and aretic symptoms or a combination of the various syndromes.

Kestenberg (1952) studied a 13½ year old schizophrenic girl. She was slow, lazy, and a poor eater from early childhood; her conversations were flat, and she gave the impression of a hebephrenic. Sue's mother demanded that Sue keep aloof from the rest of the world. Sue gave up her basic ego functions and lowered her intelligence level in order to fit into the type of life demanded by her mother, and renounced all normal contacts with reality. Since all energy that Sue possessed was used up in complying with her mother's wishes, Sue had no more left for herself.

Wittman and Huffman (1945) studied teenage schizophrenics who ranged from 15 to 20 years old when they were classified according to reaction type. The authors suggest that parental attitudes are of tremendous importance in influencing the severity of adolescent schizophrenia.

Bender grouped schizophrenic adolescent boys in Bellevue according to the following categories:

1. Acute psychotic disturbances with the onset in adolescence. Such episodes often start with a pseudoneurotic picture or severe neurosis with phobias, acute anxiety, compulsive or obsessional thoughts, hysterical conversion symptoms, or psychosomatic features.

2. Pseudodefective or autistic boys who have been mentally ill from their earliest childhood and run a chronic course, not responding to treatment. During puberty and adolescence, there may be an increase in impulsivity, compulsivity, and aggression with erotic behavior. Some of these boys have had convulsions around the time of puberty.

3. Boys known to be schizophrenic before puberty continue into adolescence with pseudoneurotic or psychotic disorders.

4. Boys known to be schizophrenic in childhood who show a change in symptomatology in puberty and continue for a shorter or longer period with mild behavior disorders.

5. Childhood schizophrenics whose adolescence is near symptomfree, but who develop psychopathic characteristics, acting out against others with no apparent anxiety or guilt.

6. Delinquent and antisocial boys who are basically schizophrenic.

Bender feels that children who appeared nearly normal in puberty, with further development into adolescence showed definite signs of disturbance. They were unable to identify with peers, accept social ideologies or authority figures or concepts. Their impulses were not controlled nor their anxiety. Attitudes and fantasies were acted out against the immediate initiating situation. Such behavior is characterized as psychopathic until it reaches explosive degrees or a chronic state.

Since the early adolescent pattern of defenses is characterized by the suppression of anxiety with secondary symptom formation and by impulsive antisocial acting out, many disturbed adolescents look alike whether they are basically schizophrenic, mildly brain damaged, or emotionally deprived and underprivileged (see Chapter 6).

Neubauer and Steinhart (1952) described the disturbances of rhythm in biological processes such as sleeping or eating with explosive irritability. In the realm of disturbed affect adolescent schizophrenics have shown marked apathy and depression.

Sands (1956) in a study on over 100 adolescent schizophrenics noticed their difficulty in relating themselves to people. Often a retiring, socially or emotionally dull behavior suddenly changes into a state of mutism, panicky attitude, and a plethora of frightening ideas, such as depersonalization, loss of control over their own body, and alleged change of shape of hands or legs. I once treated an 18 year old boy who believed that his chest was shrinking. In some cases catatonic stupors occur, with refusal of food and homicidal or suicidal attempts, lack of continence, and compulsive, overt masturbation (Sands, 1956).

Toward a Full-Blown Adult Schizophrenia

Adolescence is a period of reorganization and reestablishment of the ego and superego. The following is from Blos (1962, pp. 173-174):

It might be helpful to define the preconditions which the ego must possess at the onset of adolescence to an appreciable degree in order to develop those qualities and functions that are specifically adolescent and that will bring about those ego transformations which result in the ego of adulthood. The essential ego achievements of the latency period are the following: (1) An increase in cathexis of inner objects (object and self-representations) with resultant automatization of certain ego functions; (2) an increasing resistivity of ego functions to regression (secondary autonomy) with a consequent expansion of the nonconflictual sphere on the ego; (3) the formation of a self-critical ego which increasingly complements the functions of the superego, so that the regulation of self-esteem has reached a degree of independence from the environment; (4) reduction of the expressive use of the whole body and increase in the capacity for verbal expression in isolation from motor activity; (5) mastery of the environment through the learning of skills and the use of secondary process thinking as a means to reduce tension. The reality principle stabilizes the use of postponement and anticipation in the pursuit of pleasure.

All adolescents face serious problems of adjustment to their future sexual, occupational, and civic roles. The adolescent, being neither child nor adult, struggles with the problems of sex and age role identification.

This identification is closely related to the reshaping of the superego in adolescence. The superego is usually formed in the phallic stage (in hypervectorial cases even earlier) and faces new challenges during adolescence. The initial identification with the parental figures is exposed in adolescence to contesting influences, stemming from idealized parental images which are challenged by other heroes, presented to the growing youth by history, religion, public life, entertainment, and peers. A normal adolescent goes through considerable difficulties till he finds his way in absorbing the cultural values of his society, reshaping of his superego, and forming of his own philosophy and set of values (Blos, 1962; Deutsch, 1967; Erikson, 1968; Wolman, 1949, 1951, 1970b).

These difficulties can be unsurmountable for a hypervectorial individual. The increased pressures of his infantile, maternal, dictatorial superego may come to a point where any activity is believed to be wrong. A severe rigidity and tense passivity may lead into a catatonic stupor at this age. I have seen several catatonics whose childhood history was a story of a severe obsessive-compulsive neurosis. In the socially regulated patterns of behavior of school years and the latency period, the neurotic ego protective mechanisms kept the ego going without major setbacks. But when the human body grows and changes rapidly and the adolescent faces new social roles and expectations, the existing safety valves may prove inadequate and a flood may start. This is probably the reason for the frequent onset of manifest schizophrenia in adolescence in individuals who have been hypervectorial neurotics or latent psychotics in childhood.

This is exactly what happened to Susanne. She was obedient, conforming, and conscientious, a good student in school and a perfect child at home. Even her highly demanding mother admitted that "Susie tried to be good." Adolescence was the beginning of her manifest psychosis. Her father kept telling her all boys are bad and hurt girls, and her mother caught her reading a love story and called her "dirty." Susie began to fail in school and avoid people. She complained of headaches and "panic" feelings. At 17 the girl locked herself up in her room and refused to go out. She feared snakes, snails, turtles, frogs, and mice. When her parents told her that none of these animals were around in the apartment, she whispered, "I am also afraid of you." A few days later she said that people were watching her and the blinds of her room must be shut. For a few weeks she continued to whisper, till she became mute and immobile in a catatonic stupor.

The underlying mechanism of this case is the same as described before. The manifest onset was in this case precipitated by her incestuous "crush" on her father, who did not allow her to see other men, and her overt Oedipal hate to mother.

The downward adjustment process leads in adolescence toward one of the four types or syndromes of the full-fledged schizophrenia.

A 16 year old girl was developing obvious signs of paranoid schizophrenia. She had always been a shy, withdrawn, and over conscientious neurotic. Now when the growing destrudo pressure became unbearable, she began to have paranoid delusions, accusing her father of sexual advances and her mother of efforts to get rid of her.

The high-strung 16 year old girl began to complain of headaches. She had several crying spells and feelings of unreality. Apparently her symptoms were indicative of the simple deterioration syndrome.

Another patient, a scientifically minded, latent schizophrenic 15 year old boy began to make incongruous statements and illogical comments. He also laughed at the most improper times and places. He had always been a shy, withdrawn, very tense boy with several behavioral peculiarities. He had been collecting birds, studying astronomy, and was often inattentive or overattentive. When the pressure grew stronger, his downward adjustment led into hebephrenia.

A latent schizophrenic may turn in adolescence into a manifest schizophrenic at a slight frustration. The tensions created by biopsychological and sociopsychological factors are strong enough to cause temporary emotional upheavals in adolescents who develop later into adjusted adults. For a latent schizophrenic, these tensions may prove disastrous.

CHAPTER 5

Preschizophrenic Neuroses

1. SCHIZO-TYPE CHILDHOOD DISORDERS

The Idea of Continuum

Not every child exposed to schizogenic or schizophrenogenic (these two terms are used interchangeably) family life must become schizophrenic. The hypervectorial type of deterioration does not necessarily present a continuum. As explained in previous chapters, some children become severely psychotic at the onset of their life before they are given the opportunity to develop the most elementary parts of their mental apparatus. These pseudo-amentive children resemble plants that have been destroyed before they had any chance for growth and development. Next come the autistic, then the symbiotic, then the aretic syndromes in order of decreasing severity.

One can present adult mental disorders in a continuum of neurosis, character neurosis, latent psychosis, manifest psychosis, and dementive state (Wolman, 1965b). However, not all patients must go through all or some of these stages. When the noxious elements are powerful and act in very early childhood, they may prevent any growth and the patient starts in a dementive state such as pseudo-amentive schizophrenia.

In many schizogenic families the firstborn gets the brunt of parental "love," and the second child, less exposed to parental emotions, may develop comparatively good reality testing with some degree of overdependence on maternal approval. In a testing situation a five year old bright boy had one answer to all questions, "I ask my Mommy." However, with a little encouragement and insistence, the child passed the intelligence test very well.

Undoubtedly this child was what one might have called symbiotic, but he was not psychotic. He possesesed good reality testing and he was sensible and well-behaved. The main reason the child was brought to the office was that he was a shy, oversensitive, and rather passive child who rarely volunteered for any activities and shied away from other children. He was a daydreamer, afraid to do things on his own, overattached to his mother, and reluctant to join the other children in play and work. Yet this child, believed to be mentally retarded, was neither retarded nor psychotic. He was a hypervectorial neurotic, somewhat of the neurasthenic type.

I saw this boy in a single consultation and I do not know what happened to him later in life. Whether he improved or deteriorated depends on a variety of factors. Obviously not all individuals exposed to schizogenic (or schizophrenogenic) interindividual relations become full schizophrenics. Some arrest at a neurotic level. It is exceedingly important not to confuse the hypervectorial schizotype infantile neurosis with a full schizophrenic psychosis, as will be emphasized in Chapter 7 on psychotherapy.

Despert presented the issue with convincing clarity. She compared (1955) four cases of obsessive-compulsive neurosis with two cases of childhood psychosis. Despert noticed that schizophrenic children show lack of contact with reality, impairment of abstract thinking, and a strong guilt reaction in the obsessive-compulsives. She interpreted the preoccupation with death as a wish for self-punishment. Baldwin (1955) based differential diagnosis on the child's early life history. Disturbances in sleep, vomiting, refusal to take solid food, diarrhea, respiratory diseases, speech disorders, etc., were signs of psychosis.

The main ego function, reality testing, is little if at all damaged in neurosis, whereas in schizophrenia "it is badly shattered." The essence of the infantile hypervectorial neurosis is the desperate struggle of the child to please and protect his protectors. The overdemanding attitude of mother fosters a too early formation of superego. Normally there are only superego forerunners at the anal stage, related to conformity with the anal training. In these children, as explained before, the superego is formed very early.

The hypervectorial neurotic child is a child who has *surrendered to the demanding mother without surrendering his ego*. Probably mother's pressure was not too harsh, and the child could accept it at a cost of a slight distortion of reality by rationalization. Instead of the complete autistic or symbiotic surrender or the aretic acting out of destrudo, the neurotic child developed phobias, compulsions, and other ego protective symptoms.

The precocious superego dominates the personality of the hyper-vectorial neurotic child. The child introjects mother's image; her wishes become his law, and her criticism is the most important thing to avoid. The neurotic infant becomes a "model child." Later in his life he may suffer a psychotic breakdown, but the downward proc-ess starts much earlier.

The Superego

Normal mothers are vectorial and give unconditional love. Schiz-ogenic mothers attach strings to their love; they demand unreserved devotion and unlimited gratefulness on the part of the child. It is as if mother were saying (some mothers do say), "Either you do what I tell you and renounce your own wishes and desires, or you are a bad child." A hypervectorial neurotic child is a child whose superego is strong enough to make the child conform to mother's wishes without destroying his ego.

The overgrowth of superego is one of the most important aspects of personality deformation in all schizophrenic disorders. Wexler correctly observed that "a primitive, archaic, and devastatingly prim-itive superego plays an important role, along with urgent instinctual demands, in producing schizophrenic disorganization" (Wexler, 1952, p. 185). Also Hartmann (1953) in accordance with his "neutralization" theory, stressed the role played by archaic super-ego in schizophrenics. The *overgrowth of superego* is undoubtedly one of the outstanding features in the formation of schizophrenia (Wolman, 1957; 1966).

The study of childhood schizophrenia sheds additional light on the role played by the superego. In hypervectorial neurosis the re-pression is done by the ego in the service of superego. When the defense mechanisms fail, the quiet, subdued child may become overtly psychotic with an aretic-type acting out.

The description of the symptoms of childhood neurosis undoubt-edly could take up a separate volume, for as mentioned above, the facts of maturation and development through interaction (condition-ing and cathexis) complicate the clinical picture.

Symptoms

One of the outstanding symptoms common to all types of hyper-vectorial disorders is the *constant fear of and preoccupation with death*. This fear may be hidden and expressed in a disguised, often in a pseudo-philosophical way. Some children ask questions about the future of the earth, mankind, rivers, or stars. They worry about the age of their parents. Some worry about where the water goes from the pipes. All of them fear change in the daily life routine; moving to another city or to new neighborhood is a frightening experience to them.

As mentioned before, the child's insistence on sameness is an expression of that fear. As long as things go on in the usual way, life continues. A change represents a threat to the continuation of life, for unpredictable things may happen that frighten the child. As long as things do not change, the child feels he has everything under his hypervectorial control. Quite often in schizogenic families the child assumes dictatorial control over the actions of his parents. Of course this rule is frequently interrupted by temper tantrums in which parents and children alike participate.

The diversity in symptoms of the hypervectorial neurotic in children depends on their particular life history and interaction patterns within their families. Some children have nervous twitches; some experience eating difficulties, nauseas, regurgitation, even anorexias. Eating difficulties have often been created by overanxious mothers who by forcing food on the child have tried to compensate for their guilt feelings. Many of these children are overweight; they have overeaten to please mother, to show her how good they are. When mother's anxieties are not particularly related to feeding, the child has no problems with food. If mother suffers nauseas, the child may identify himself with her. If mother is overanxious or oversolicitous in putting the child to sleep, the child is very tense lest he not fall asleep immediately. An adolescent patient recalled how he cried in his little bed because he was not yet asleep; in latency and puberty he experienced panicky feelings, whenever he failed to have the $8\frac{1}{2}$ hours prescribed by his mother. Other children cannot fall asleep for worrying; they know that mother and father will start their routine fights immediately after putting the children to bed.

The hypervectorial neurotic child is often immaculately clean, orderly, and conforming. Sometimes his conformity and perfect behavior mollify mother's attitude, and the child grows into adulthood as a vectorial neurotic without psychotic deterioration.

The other anal traits, such as parsimony and obstinacy, are no less significant in the formation of schizotype personality traits. Parsimony is the fear of loss of what one has. Hypervectorials are poor losers; they cannot part with animate or inanimate love objects. They invest so much libido in their love objects that separation is always a heavy loss and a severe blow to them. Obstinacy is the same in a more symbolic way; it is the fear of losing the ideas one possesses. One step down in the process of deterioration, and the child develops ideas of reference.

In early childhood the clinical picture is dominated by the fear of separation from mother, that is, the fear of independence and growing up. The child is frightened whenever he is left alone or when asked to do things by himself. He may continue infantile ways of eating, refuse to dress himself, and be overly passive in order to perpetuate maternal overprotection. The reader is reminded that the refusal of an adult catatonic to take care of himself is an invitation to others to take care of him; it is a regression into the symbiotic childhood syndrome (Wolman, 1966).

Hypervectorial neurotic children often develop psychosomatic symptoms. Hypochondriac complaints may have already started in the preschool age, although they usually do not begin until the school age and latency period. In almost all of the cases I have seen, the child's somatic complaints have been related to parental hypochondriasis or their parents' true illness. These parents had used their own true or imaginary aches and pains to gain sympathy and support from their marital partners. When frustrated in their instrumentalism, they turned toward the child and tried to get comfort from the child. Some of these mothers eagerly told the child how strong, beautiful, and healthy they were before they bore the child. One mother said bluntly to the child, "You hurt me, you almost killed me during birth, and now you're finishing up your job of killing your mother." Some mothers had headaches, backaches, toothaches, heartburn, nausea, vomiting spells, and blamed all these on the child, saying, "You made your mother sick."

Many hypervectorial children are used as an "organ of parental hypochondriasis." Kanner (1960, p. 616) described a case of a little girl whose "bowels had become her mother's organ of hypochondriacal agitation."

When the children entered the phallic period and face the Oedipal complex, many of them masturbate excessively and some act out their sexual impulses publicly, touching and looking on, and thus coming pretty close to hebephrenic behavior with no inhibitions. Typically, hypervectorial neurotic children develop severe repression, denial, and displacement mechanisms. Their sex identification is never too clear, and there is no sublimation of sex or hostility, but there is most often a powerful repression of both. Most of these children fear sex and hostility, and they neither masturbate nor fight.

In cases when the parental pressures are mild, the child may grow into a neurotic school child and later into an adult neurotic. In some cases, when the child receives systematic therapy or experiences friendly social contacts, ego compensatory symptoms may develop.

2. OBSESSIVE-COMPULSIVE CHILDHOOD NEUROSIS

The Superego

The hypervectorial neurotic child is a child whose ego has remained relatively intact despite the instrumentalism of his parents. Although parental instrumentalism has forced the child to embark upon the road of hypervectorialism that might ultimately lead to schizophrenia, the child's ego has received some libido compensation. Thus, he is neurotic and may never become a manifest psychotic. Yet the main elements of the hypervectorial disorder are easily distinguishable even in childhood neurosis. Because of parental instrumentalism and the interparental strife, the child views his parents as *weak,* i.e., unable to protect him. As a result, he feels forced to *protect his protectors.* He fears that, should he fail, they will die and he will be forsaken and doomed to death. While giving emotional support to his parents (object hypercathexis), the child impoverishes his own resources and is unable to exercise adequate self-cathexis. The impoverished ego develops a series of ego protective symptoms.

One can distinguish several symptomatological patterns in the childhood hypervectorial neurosis. One of them is self-sacrifice, conformity, renunciation of pleasure principle, and early development of a distorted reality principle. The hypervectorial neurotic child accepts toilet training early and perfectly and develops bowel and bladder control with a tendency to constipation and infrequent urination.

Under the threat of losing his hypercathected love object, the mother, the child introjects her image already at the anal stage. This leads to a precocious formation of a despotic, rigid, and over-demanding superego. An early development of superego, as several authors and especially Melanie Klein (1957) have emphasized, is essential for the development of the obsessive-compulsive neurosis in childhood.

The neurotic child is frequently a model child, obedient, complying, reserved, and displaying excellent manners. His is the "constricted" type of personality so often found in obsessive-compulsive neurotics. In the hypervectorial childhood neurosis, the main symptoms reflect repression of hostile impulses. The children are anxious, often hypochondriac, and some of them develop phobias and compulsions. As a result of the struggle of the ego against both id and superego, the child is constantly tense, overalert, and anxious. He feels guilty no matter what he does, because he can never satisfy his nagging mother nor her image incorporated in his own severe superego.

Compulsive Traits

An investigation of the characteristics of obsessive-compulsive behavior isolated four traits, namely, rigidity, compulsive activity, moral obligation, and loss of contact with reality (Shapiro, 1962). Rigidity refers to the persistence of a type of behavior which is irrelevant or absurd.

Although the attention of an obsessive-compulsive is not totally restricted, as is characteristic of brain-damaged patients, he does not enjoy the freedom of movement which "normal" individuals experience. Rorschach responses support this fact. Rather than viewing the whole inkblot, they pick out fine and precise details in much the same way as they carry on their daily activities.

Narrowness, intensity, and fixation of attention belong to the symptoms of obsessive-compulsive neurosis. Many obsessive-compulsive individuals refer to their lives as well-run machines which are aiming in one direction and are incapable of changing that direction. Individuals of this nature do not possess the feelings of free will or sense of autonomy. "For the obsessive-compulsive person, everything involves a special sense of trying" (Shapiro, p. 54). Every activity performed by obsessive-compulsive children involves an effort; such a child feels that he must do a certain thing, and a special effort is necessary. The compulsive child believes that his behavior and the intensive energy that drives it are not a product of his own free will; he attributes them to the will of a higher authority. Thus he often uses the term, "I should," perceived as a sense of moral obligation. The phrases "I should" and "I must" are quite noticeable in the speech of the compulsive. "Experiencing a continuous pressure that feels separate from and alien to his own wishes is the very condition that allows the compulsive to feel the presence of a command under which he can serve" (Shapiro, p. 56).

Childhood obsessions similar to those of adults have been observed by Michaux and Dugas (1959), who have divided the obsessional neurosis into three categories: (1) obsessions proper, which are defined as constantly recurring thoughts of an irrational nature; (2) phobias, or fears attached to habits and objects; (3) and compulsions, which they describe as fears of carrying out inappropriate compulsive activities, such as crying in church or laughing at a funeral. Apparently, obsessive neurosis in childhood is characterized by the three components of anxiety, uncertainty, insecurity, and indecision.

The obsessive child displays similar rigidity to that observed in adult obsessives; there is, however, a tendency for the child to confine his attention to actions and ideas related to his desire to attain perfection. The obsessive child retains feelings of incompleteness unless his compulsive acts are executed. "Their writing is immaculate and they spend a great deal of time arranging objects in an immutable order" (Michaux and Dugas, p. 7). They say their prayers over and over again for fear of not having said them perfectly.

The obsessive child often wonders about his own body, and about himself and his interpersonal relations (Do I love my mother? Am

I myself? Is this me who is thinking?). He puts his parents to the test to determine their love for him. "Very often the only manifestations of obsessional neurosis in children is limited to difficulties in their expression" (Michaux and Dugas, p. 8).

The young child is incapable of being aware of his obsessions. Most of his compulsive actions, which are reactions to obsessive fears, are carried out because the child thinks that they are magical and if constantly exerecised will bring about a release from these fears.

The authors have emphasized three problems in the diagnosis of obsessive children. The first is that tics, which are characteristic of this disorder, do not necessarily result from it. Second, all obsessions are not synonymous with obsessive neurosis. There may be scattered fears in normal children which do not occur regularly and thus are not neurotic. Finally, not all obsessive symptoms are neurotic; some are epileptic and encephalitic syndromes.

The severity of obsessive-compulsive neurosis depends upon the child's relative tolerance to stress and also upon the amount or degree of stress he receives from the environment. The consequences of these disorders may range anywhere from uncomfortable behavioral symptoms, which are bothersome to the individual or others around him, up to self- or other-inflicted injury.

The role of the parent-child factor in the causation of childhood obsessions was demonstrated by Schmidelberg (1948) in the form of obsessional inability to make decisions. Interparental strife makes the child feel guilty at having to take the side of one parent against the other. In some of these cases the obsessional indecision has been removed by the patient himself by his turning to an obsessional decision, and thus producing a partial relief from neurotic symptoms.

Social Relations

Not all hypervectorial neurotic children are socially withdrawn, but all of them display certain peculiarities in interaction with their peers. Children of this age tend to be clannish and form closed groups and cliques, but hypervectorial children are even more choosy about their friends. Some of them shy away from other children who are (according to mother) rowdy and dirty or belong to

another race, creed, or ethnic group. When, however, a hypervectorial neurotic child forms a friendship with another child, it usually involves a great deal of attachment, devotion, and loyalty. An
intelligent neurotic child may become a leader of his class or play
group. He will be devoted to his role, very conscientious, but also
demanding and even dictatorial. While he himself adheres strictly
to the rules, he may try to impose them on the other members of
the group.

Some obsessive-compulsive children shun leadership and other
social contacts. They fear they will be blamed for shortcomings or
inadequacies and prefer to stay loyal followers. They may worry
that they may lose their friends and get hurt and they avoid proximity out of fear of rejection.

Obsessive-compulsive children easily accept authority and are,
as a rule, compliant and conforming students. Many of them are
model students in the lower grades, where conformity with teacher's
demands is rewarded.

School years usually witness the onset of many obsessive-compulsive symptoms. Rarely do these symptoms start before the age
of six, and mostly they start later in the latency period. These children are "overconscientious, shy, pedantic, punctilious, painstak-
ingly addicted to minute orderliness and symmetry" (Kanner, 1960,
p. 621). The obsessive-compulsive symptoms serve as a barrier
against the unresolved Oedipal wishes. Observation of obsessive-
compulsive children and longitudinal studies on adult schizophrenics who were neurotics in their childhood shed light on the origin
of compulsive behavior that has in all cases served the main purpose of *warding off sexual and aggressive impulses.*

Self-Control

The obsessive-compulsive child is forced to adhere strictly to
parental request under the threat of being blamed for whatever
troubles his parents might have had. Absolute conformity, strict
routine, and rigidity seem to be the best protection against doing
wrong that may upset the existing order in which the hypercathected
parents are somehow able to survive. The child is afraid of changes
for they may be fraught with new dangers. When mother comes
home late or father is delayed in town, the child cannot fall asleep.

One child developed a complete ritual before going to bed to ward off his "bad thoughts," his desire to look under mother's dress.

One of the main reasons for forming compulsive action patterns is the *fear of losing self-control.* Many children worry that they may lose control of their bowels. Some are afraid they may be tempted to masturbate. Others are afraid that they may get indigestion and vomit. Since all of these things have been always perceived by mother as an intentional defiance of her orders and an intentionally malicious act of the ungrateful child ("Look what you have done to your mother"), the child may have difficulty in falling asleep, fear to go places, fear to eat, and have many other phobias.

Any change is a threat and challenge to the child's aspiration for mastery over himself and his environment. The child's displaced fears turn into a series of taboos, restrictions, rituals, and compulsive acts. One little boy developed *délire de toucher,* while another had a compulsion to touch. One girl was afraid to go out (agoraphobia), while another was afraid to stay indoors (claustrophobia). The choice of symptoms is never coincidental. It is always a product of specific pressures and threats, reflecting the actual happenings in the child's interaction with his parents.

From Neurosis to Psychosis

Many obsessive-compulsive children develop paranoid ideas resembling those of paranoid schizophrenia. The hypervectorial, overdemanding superego is severely critical of one's hostile and sexual impulses and the hard-pressed ego joins the superego in repressing the unconscious impulses, forming obsessive-compulsive defenses. These neurotic defenses are ego-protective.

Should these defenses fail, further deterioration may occur, leading either toward paranoid or catatonic schizophrenia in a gradual or sudden development of paranoid or catatonic ego deficiency symptoms. In several cases, both paranoid and obsessional mechanisms operate in a combination that leads to latent schizophrenia without apparent personality disintegration. Most catatonic patients I worked with had an obsessive-compulsive childhood history (Wolman, 1966).

Apparently, obsessive-compulsive neurosis is the first step on the road of the downward adjustment in hypervectorial disorders (cf. Chapter 2). The same dynamic factors act in the obsessive-compulsive neurosis as in a full schizophrenic, both in childhood and adulthood. In all hypervectorial disorders there is the object hypercathected attitude to parents, fear of own hostile impulses, and overgrown superego.

A case described by Bender may serve as an illustration in support of this theory (1954, p. 125):

> Mae was a twelve year old girl . . . admitted to the hospital because of her refusal to go to school for the previous term. She stated that she did not want to leave her mother alone. She had obsessive thoughts of her mother being killed and being run down by automobiles. She had developed a touching compulsion in order to ward off "bad luck" from her mother.

Another patient, 12 year old Frances, had obsessional ideas of a sexual nature centered around her mother, her mother's genitals, etc. Bender remarked that "the importance of the parent-child relationship in all these cases was apparent. Precipitatory events, when present, seemed to touch off deeper seated problems in relation to the emotional attitude of the patient toward his parents" (*ibid.*, p. 127).

Bender, like many other workers, stressed the aggressive and destructive tendencies present in the symptoms of the obsessive-compulsive neurosis. In the cases described by Bender, the psychotic onset was between five and eight years of age.

My interpretation of the nature of the obsessive-compulsive syndrome of hypervectorial childhood neurosis is supported by a review of one of Kanner's (1960) cases involving a six year old obsessive-compulsive girl. Kanner's case strikingly resembles my description of schizogenic family relationships (Chapter 1). The father had little contact with the child, and the mother was nagging, demanding, and did not allow the child to leave the house because of "bad" children in the vicinity. The mother's concepts of "right" and "wrong" were hammered into the little girl's head, and the little girl was perpetually criticized and made aware of her inadequacies. Maternal preoccupation with the child's feeding and bowel movements created problems of anorexia and constipation.

The differential diagnosis between manifest childhood schizophrenia and hypervectorial childhood neurosis is not always easy. Despert (1955) stressed the fact that a neurotic child is aware of the irrationality of his experiences and fantasy distortion, and that in a psychotic child there is a break with reality and impairment of intellectual function. However, Weil (1953) and Wolman (1966) found obsessive-compulsive symptoms, such as sleep disturbances, hypochondriac complaints, etc., in both neurosis and psychosis.

There are, as a rule, fewer behavioral fluctuations in neurosis than in manifest psychosis. The manifestly schizophrenic child acts sometimes like a neurotic, sometimes almost normal; the neurotic child, however, does not act like a psychotic. Ekstein and others (1954, 1969) pointed to the stronger ego of the neurotic child, which protects primary processes. Some workers have not noticed the continuum in all hypervectorial disorders, while my observations point to this continuum (Wolman, 1957, 1965b). The obsessive-compulsive symptoms in childhood and adulthood are not opposites; they are distinct levels of the same disorder, distinguished by the fighting or failing ego, respectively.

As long as the child is aware of the irrationality of his obsessive thoughts and compulsive acts, he is neurotic, no matter how strange his thoughts and acts. As long as the child knows that his fantasies are fantasies, he is not yet psychotic. As long as his ego does reality testing and more or less controls his impulses, he is neurotic. When the ego fails, psychosis starts.

Anna Freud's summary presented at the Twenty-Fourth International Psychoanalytic Congress (1966) may well serve as a summary of our discussion of the obsessive-compulsive neurosis in childhood. This neurosis represents a variety of clinical pictures bordering on the one hand on the nearly normal, ego syntonic states, and on the other leading to schizoid status and full schizophrenic psychosis. The varied symptomatology of obsessional neurosis depends on a multitude of etiologic factors, such as the relative role of father or mother as main targets of the child's hostile wishes, the choice of particular defense mechanisms, and so on.

3. CHILDHOOD PHOBIAS

Phobic reactions are one of the choice symptoms in childhood neurosis of the hypervectorial type. The insecure parents expect from the child more than the child can give to them, and the "overdemanded" child resents his parents, but their self-styled martyrdom block his normal outlets of anger. When his mother and father fight one another and the child fears losing one or both of them, he becomes afraid that his hostility may hurt them.

When this conflict is not so severe as to destroy the child's personality, the child's ego applies neurotic defenses. One type of such defenses are the above-described obsessive-compulsive symptoms; phobias are another type. Phobias use defense mechanisms of displacement and withdrawal, thus blocking direct outlets for anger. Whenever these defenses fail, the phobic hypervectorial neuroticism leads into a fullblown schizophrenia (Wolman, 1966).

Research work conducted independently seems to support the above-described explanation. For instance, Colm (1959) found that the mother's anxiety is felt by the child as emotional desertion. When mother's anxiety becomes too intense and too severe and the mother's defenses against it are too confusing to the child, the child responds in a neurotic way. The child will tend to comply compulsively with his mother's defensive ways of coping with her anxieties, and his compulsive defenses aim at controlling his own panic and resentment.

In phobias the child displaces and symbolizes his anxiety, producing hostility. The phobic child does not allow himself to be aware of his hostile feelings toward his parents. Instead he withdraws and represses his conflict. He takes a sort of refuge in a phobia, displacing his fright and hate onto an outside object and avoiding the frightening feeling that he wishes his mother dead.

Parents of the phobic type are vacillating and overcontrolling at the same time. They disagree between themselves in the handling of their children, and most often no consistent standards of behavior are set for the child. These parents are obviously unable to guide the child, and the child senses not only that the parents are anxious and unsure but that by conforming to the same rigid rules he offers reassurance to his parents.

The difference between parents of phobic and of schizophrenic children is a matter of degree. There is the self-conflicting, "double-bind" talk (Bateson et al., 1956), and the talking does not correspond to what the parents really feel. Parental talk is anxiety-ridden and evidently contradicts what they unconsciously convey to the child. The phobic child senses the intense anxiety and hidden hostility of his parents, and is only utterly confused by their attempts to cover their true feelings by verbose declarations of self-sacrificing love. Most of these parents are unaware of the fact that *they unconsciously want love to be given to them by the child, while consciously they believe that they give love to the child.* The child *cannot trust the parents to help him,* as he needs to be helped, but feels that he must reassure them and become their protector (cf. Chapter 2). The phobic and the schizophrenic child feels that he is alone despite so much talk about love, protection, and security. Parents of phobic and other hypervectorial children live their own unresolved childhood needs vicariously, utterly unable to see the needs of the child. The child, frustrated in his normal instrumental need to be loved and cared for, and forced into hypervectorial, caring attitude toward his parents, hates them intensely and fears that his hate may hurt them. Hence the hypervectorial vicious cycle: hate for the parents—guilt—hate for himself—hate for the parents. He constantly feels guilty for hating his weak and seductive parents; since his parents cannot be trusted to control him and the situation, he must assume control, and he develops ritualistic compulsions or phobic symbols. His hate for his parents causes him to hate himself, and his phobias become thus a partial self-punishment.

Conditioning

Wolpe and Rachman (1960) believe that phobias are conditioned anxiety (fear) reactions. Any "neutral" stimulus, simple or complex, that happens to make an inpact on an individual at about the time that fear reaction is evoked acquires the ability to evoke fear consequently. If the fear at the original conditioning situation is of high intensity or if the conditioning is many times repeated, the conditioned fear persists in a way characteristic of neurotic fear. The fear reactions to stimuli resembling the conditioned stimulus may become generalized.

Rachman and Costello (1961) hypothesized that neurotic symptoms are learned patterns of behavior which for some reason or another are unadaptive. Neurotic behavior patterns persist paradoxically, because they are unpleasant. Having acquired an unpleasant association and reaction to a particular stimulus or situation, the child tends to avoid exposure to these noxious circumstances. Such an avoidance may become symbolized and phobic.

School Phobia

One of the most frequent symptoms is school phobia. The term school phobia was first used by Johnson (1941) as a description of symptoms characterized by intense terror associated with school (Johnson et al., 1941). Wallinga (1959, p. 258) describes it thus:

School phobia is a clearly defined emotional disturbance occurring most frequently in children 6-10 years. It is characterized by an intense anxiety which is first related to leaving for school in the morning. The anxiety commonly appears with increasing anxiety at the beginning of each school year or after vacation. Often the child has been ill for a few weeks, or has experienced an emotional upset. He is overwhelmed with anxiety when expected to return to school. This feeling may be recognized by nightmares, nausea, etc. The particular physical complaint is often a reflection of a similar symptom in one of the parents whom the child has been worrying about.

The intrafamilial interaction of phobic children closely resembles that in schizophrenic families. The mothers of children with school phobia profess a self-sacrificing attitude. They are restrictive and controlling, but they waver between strictness and leniency. "Lurking behind the wish to do everything possible for her child is her deep-felt uncertainty about her confidence as a mother" (Waldfogel et al., 1957, p. 757). One mother gave up breast feeding her child because she felt it did not get enough to eat, yet the child grew at a normal rate. "It is this feeling of inadequacy in her maternal role which is basic to the mother's own anxiety at separation" (*ibid.*, p. 757).

According to Davidson (1961) the mothers are perfectionistic, "having an idealized picture of what constitutes a good mother, and feel guilty for not having attained this goal. They expect perfect love and compliance from the child, and are hurt when they do not get it and often look upon this as evidence of their own failure" (Davidson, 1961, p. 281).

Talbot (1957) found that the fathers have never been emancipated from their own families, both parents and siblings. Agras (1958) found that of eight fathers, three drank, one had been hospitalized for a psychotic depressive episode, three were passive, ineffectual, and poor providers, and one had deserted his family.

School phobia is like other phobias of childhood, but the anxiety in this instance is shifted from its basic source to the school. Practically all research workers trace the origins of school phobia to the child's *fear of being separated from his mother*. Mothers of phobic children see narcissistic gratification through the child. When the child is a girl, the mother identifies herself with the little girl's appearance, intelligence, or achievement. The male child may be used by the mother for erotic gratification, the mother often becoming involved in bodily contact under the guise of affection and playfulness. Even when the mother is angry with the child, she does not withdraw her affection but is more apt to "reason" with him, a procedure which usually consists of a "soliloquacious" speech comprised of nagging and pleading. Mothers of hypervectorial children rarely resort to physical punishment, and whenever they do they usually apologize to the child.

The mothers of phobic children display a peculiar dependence-subservience to the child. They tend to sacrifice their own need and comforts and act in an exceedingly overprotective manner. These mothers try to protect the child from pain, shock, and frustration.

The fathers, because of their anxiety concerning their sexual identification, fail in defining their parental role. Many fathers of phobic children are involved with the problems of child care, as if trying to prove that they can handle the children better than the mothers, thus undermining in the mothers their already shaky feeling of maternal adequacy (Waldfogel et al., 1957).

The Role of Parents

According to Goldberg (1953) at least one parent of a phobic child had a marked personality difficulty and unresolved conflict, "most mothers and some fathers still being involved on an infantile level with their own families in adult life. Over one-third of the mothers were controlling, two-thirds of the fathers were passive and inadequate" (Goldberg, 1953, p. 244).

Immaturity leads to marital discord, which in turn may lead to the parental cause of school phobia. Goldberg (1953) found that many of the parents maintained that they remained together only for the sake of the child. Some wives refused sexual relations with their husbands and slept with the child. Some spouses remained so involved with their own parents that their marriage played only a minor part in their lives. Their marriage, which lacked emotional gratification for the mother, caused the mother to turn to the child, who had to be both his mother's child and lover. The child is often resented "as a hostage by whose presence the mother was trapped" (Eisenberg, 1957, p. 215). This hostility on the part of the mother leads to guilt feelings and, as a result, to overprotection.

The peculiar mother-child relationship demonstrated by phobic children resembles the umbilical cord that pulls at both ends (Eisenberg, 1957). The mother is ambivalent towards the child, and the child in turn is ambivalent towards the mother. The mother is overprotective to the child, and the child in self-defense fights for independence from the mother. The child's striving for independence adds to her feeling of rejection and to such statements as "After all I gave her" (Eisenberg, 1957, p. 715).

The mothers of phobic children need to feel that they are needed. The child's attempt to be independent threatens the mother and increases her neurotic anxiety. Usually, the mother blames the child for her troubles, instilling in the child the fear of expressing his own normal aggressive impulses.

Some children exploit the mother's desire for their dependence upon her; such a child gains dictatorial powers over his mother and often father. The child, torn by guilt feelings, needs to be near his mother and avoids school, but by staying home he does not permit his mother to leave him even for a short while.

Under normal circumstances a child wishes to free himself gradually from mother's protection and establish his own individuality. But the inconsistency of the parents of phobic children, and their shifting from overindulgent to overpunitive attitudes, does not allow the child to gain enough security to achieve the needed independence. "The child's reaction to the parent's infantile and unpredictable behavior is the feeling of a lack of support" (Talbot, 1957).

This feeling on the part of the child that the mother wishes him to regress and remain dependent explains the fact that school phobia often develops after the child has been ill and bedridden. Physical illness increases anxiety and makes dependence on the mother real and justified. A sick child tends to regress temporarily to an earlier level of dependence upon his mother, but in schizogenic families this regression is fostered and perpetuated. According to Coolidge et al. (1957), pp. 297-208):

The central conflict revolves around a symbolic tie to the mother. The increasing external pressure and the consequent sense of inadequacy produced feelings of helplessness, which in turn increased the yearning for dependence and protection from the mother, strengthening the regressive tendencies. The fears of helplessness are partly counteracted by a pervasive and all consuming need for control.

The phobic child tries to inhibit his aggressive and libidinal impulses, which are directed at one or both parents. Sometimes the hostile feelings become overwhelming, and the ensuing feeling of guilt makes separation from the mother impossible. "By her successive preoccupation with her child's welfare and her inability to set limits effectively, the mother feeds the child's narcissism and omnipotent fantasies. The child becomes dependent upon her for gratification and she becomes an active partner in his neurosis" (Waldfogel, Coolidge, Hahn, 1957, p. 758). The parental "inability to limit his demands, which at times assume tyrannical proportions, nurture his omnipotent fantasies, supporting the tendency toward magical thinking when the wish becomes equivalent to its realization" (Waldfogel et al., 1957, p. 759).

The normal development of the child's ego is hampered by the oppressive proximity of the parents. The child rarely has the chance to cope with a difficult situation by himself, for his parents constantly try to help and protect him.

School phobia, as any other phobia, is a *displacement* of anxiety from its original source to a substitute object and the fear of mother is displaced to a fear of teacher. As in other phobias, there is *projection* of intolerable impulses; for instance, oral aggressive fantasies may be transformed into a fear of being bitten by a dangerous animal. There is also the mechanism of *externalization* by which guilt feeling is transformed into fear of being punished by some dangerous object in the environment.

In most families with phobic children there is a profound interdependence between the child and mother, and occasionally of the child with the father; also both parents and their parents are closely interacting, with little freedom left for each individual. Frequently there is too close interdependence among relatives, and frequent visiting is customary. There is often a lack of interest in people outside the close family; most often the parents, especially mothers, have no friends outside the family.

The Death Wish

The study of phobic children and their parents may offer additional insight into the mechanics of schizophrenia in childhood. Parents of these hypervectorial neurotic children are at odds with each other and resent not being given undivided attention and unlimited love by their spouses. Thus, they turn toward the child with ambivalent feelings. On one hand, they expect to receive from the child all the love and affection they cannot receive from their marital partner. This love-demanding attitude is often seductive in a hetero- or homosexual way; it is, at the same time, somewhat submissive, as if the parent were fighting for the last chance to be loved by someone.

As was explained in Chapter 2, these efforts are doomed to fail. The victories are short-lived, and defeats are frequent and painful. Many fathers who have had sexual relations with their preadolescent daughters complain to me that their daughters are "ungrateful" when the daughters finally turn them down and rebel against being used by their fathers. Practically all mothers of schizophrenic children complain about "ungrateful" children who do not reciprocate their mother's "sacrifice." Frustration breeds hostility, and the ultimate goal of hostile feeling is the annihilation of those who frustrate.

Childhood phobia is not a separate clinical entity. Practically all schizophrenic children have phobias. Some of them deteriorate further, and their phobias are transformed into paranoid structures and delusions. Some other children remain phobic, for their phobias, being ego protective, prevent or at least delay further deterioration, depending on a variety of noxious and compensatory factors in the child's environment.

All schizophrenic children are preoccupied with death, and many of them talk often about death. Death fascinates them; they fear and relish terror stories in newspapers, books, television, and movies. The phobias play a significant role in this context.

The preoccupation with death has two sources, usually the parental death wish directed against the child and child's death wish directed against his parents (Davidson, 1961; Talbot, 1957; Wolman, 1957, 1966). While the parents profess great love for their child, their inevitable frustrations and difficulties with the child cause them to hate him. Some parents express it freely saying, "I wish you were never born," but most parents try to inhibit their hostile impulses. Yet occasional outbursts clearly convey the parental death wish.

A phobia may displace a childhood fear. An adolescent patient who feared cats dreamed about cats scratching her face; in free associations she recalled similar scenes from her childhood when her mother scratched her face whenever she soiled her dress playing with children. In most cases phobias hide the child's death wish directed against his mother. The pent-up resentment may break through; I have seen schizophrenic children and adolescents physically attacking members of their family. However, attacking one's own mother may deprive one of the last source of shaky protection and create unbearable guilt feelings and a psychotic state of panic. Phobia as a displacement of a death wish is anxiety reducing and, therefore, it offers the primary gain typical of the milder cases of the hypervectorial disorder.

CHAPTER 6

Differential Diagnosis

1. HISTORICAL REMARKS

As early as 1834 Friedreich made references to psychoses in childhood, and in 1845 Griesinger and Esquirol mentioned childhood disorders. In 1887, Emminghaus wrote that since children have illnesses peculiar to themselves, the mental disorders of adult life could not possibly occur in children. Maudsley, however, maintained that all adult psychoses might at times be observed in children. In 1892, Schonthal reported 10 cases of childhood psychosis.

Despite the work done in the nineteenth century, childhood psychoses were believed to be very rare. Diagnostic statements pertaining to childhood psychosis faced serious difficulties, stemming from lack of accepted criteria for diagnosing psychoses in general and the tendency to overlook symptoms peculiar to children.

In 1905, DeSanctis introduced the term "dementia praecocissima" for cases occurring in very early life as opposed to those cases occurring around puberty, and reported several cases starting as early as the fourth year. Similar reports then appeared in the French, Italian, German, and Swiss literature. In subsequent years, however, dementia praecocissima was believed to include a great many pathologic conditions such as schizophrenia, encephalitis, and organic brain diseases. Weygandt and Heller wrote at length on what they termed "dementia infantilis" and expressed views similar to DeSanctis.

Kraepelin made only brief reference to childhood dementia praecox and stated that, in 3.5 per cent of cases in adults, the signs and symptoms could be traced back to early childhood.

In 1910, Strohmayer expressed the opinion that all the psychological disorders of adulthood with the exception of paranoia vera, arteriosclerotic psychoses, and senile dementia, can be also found in childhood.

In 1911, E. Bleuler introduced the term "schizophrenia" in order to avoid the prognostic implications of "dementia praecox." He stated that the condition may come to a standstill at any stage and that some of its symptoms may clear up to a large extent or altogether, but if it does progress, it definitely leads to dementia of a specific type. According to Bleuler, schizophrenia can start as early as in the first years of life.

Around the thirties and forties of our century, several investigators began to pay attention to psychosis in children and to study the differences between psychoses in children and in adults. Among the first to discuss this were Lurie and his associates, who concluded that "the simultaneous occurrence of an abnormal trend in the intellectual, social, and emotional development of a child without an apparent organic basis may pressage the development of a frank psychosis later in life."

Bradley (1947) proposed that the term psychosis should not be used to indicate a specific mental disease or disorder in children. "There has been, until recently, a tendency to discuss this subject in child psychology by presenting classical descriptions and groupings of adult disorders, and trying to fit certain maladjusted children into these fixed categories." Bradley defined psychosis as "a severe mental disturbance or pathological reaction pattern in which all the usual forms of adaptation to life are involved."

Schizophrenia is undoubtedly the most common childhood psychosis. According to Bradley, a schizophrenic psychosis in childhood presents a severe distortion of the entire personality, distinguished by withdrawal of interest from the enviroment. The patient seems to derive little or no real satisfaction from the ordinary events of life, and he appears to be preoccupied with his own thoughts, fantasies, and solitary activities.

Schizophrenic children show certain peculiar behavior traits, such as seclusiveness, irritability, excessive daydreaming, excessive sensitivity to being criticized, and less physical activity than would be anticipated in children of a similar age. Some of them practice monotonous, repetitive play, or rock back and forth. Speech disturbances range from mutism to unintelligible chattering. The importance of speech disorders has been emphasized further by Despert. Some of the most outstanding symptoms of adult schizophrenia were absent in many of the psychotic children examined by Bradley. Bender (1942) felt that schizophrenia in childhood offers the following diagnostic clues: (1) psychotic reactions, (2) a disturbance at every level of adaptive behavior and function, (3) a fundamental pattern of withdrawal from reality, and (4) history of difficulties in adaptation to persons and resistance to changes in the immediate environment in the early years before the onset of overt psychosis.

Many reports state that a history of a period early in life entirely free from evidence of mental illness is a fundamental characteristic of schizophrenia in childhood. In contrast to this, Bradley concludes that "the preliminary period of satisfactory adjustment does not seem essential to a good diagnosis of schizophrenia."

In 1944, Kanner introduced the term "early infantile autism" whose "characteristic features consist of a profound withdrawal from contact with people, and obsessive desire for the preservation of sameness, a skillful and even affectionate relation to objects, the retention of a pensive physiognomy, and even mutism or the kind of language which does not seem intended to serve the purpose of interpersonal communication. An analysis of this language has revealed a peculiar reversal of pronouns, neologism, metaphors, and apparently irrelevant utterances which become meaningful to the extent to which they can be traced to the patient's experiences and their emotional implications."

According to Kanner, "one can hardly speak of an insidious onset of early infantile autisms, except perhaps with reference to the first semester of life. The infants seem unusually apathetic, do not react to the approach of people, fail to assume an anticipatory posture preparatory to being picked up, and when they are picked up, do not adjust their posture to the person who holds them. They seem happiest when left alone. Persistent lack of responsiveness raises doubts about the child's hearing acuity. When it becomes obvious that hearing is not impaired, poor test performances lead to the assumption of innate feeble-mindedness. This succession of a first diagnosis of deafness and a second diagnosis of mental deficiency is almost invariably a part of the case histories of autistic children."

Bernfield (1929) feels that hallucinations may constitute a normal phenomenon in infants and young children and contends that a hungry infant hallucinates a situation in which gratification takes place. Sherman and Beverly (1924) studied a group of children whose intelligence quotients were below 100. They found that "in some children, the hallucinations were simply projections of their mental difficulty, in others a means of comprehension or explanation for their difficulty." The psychotic child, they felt, attempts to adjust by means of imagery in much the same way as the normal child uses imagery to gain wish fulfillment.

Despert (1925) studied a group of 106 children over a 10 year period at the Payne Whitney Nursery School and was unable to confirm these observations. "It can be emphatically stated that there is no evidence of true hallucinations or delusions either expressed by the children or observed by outsiders at home or at school." She also differentiated between normal and psychotic daydreaming. In the former group, daydreaming may occur suddenly during play but the child gives evidence of active mentation inwardly turned. In the psychotic child "the body tonus is depressed, the facial expression lacks animation, and there frequently appear some infantile manifestations such as sucking or chewing of the fingers."

The symptomatology depends on the age of the child. Above the tenth year level "the delusional experiences, including hallucinations, are very similar to those of adults, except for their greater simplicity and the total lack of organization and systematization of the delusional content" (Despert, 1952).

According to Robinson (1961) delusional material is absent in children. "Favored ideas are expressed in a repetitive stereotyped manner. Repetitive or compulsive motor activity often represents the evident features of illness. Hallucination is unusual, expressed in a repetitive stereotyped manner. Repetitive or compulsive motor activity often represents the evident features of illness. Hallucination is unusual, excepting in the form of momentary experiences which are associated with terror or anxiety." Robinson did not, however, finish the picture. He stated that repetitive stereotyped statements may suggest hallucinations, but one must question whether such statements are based on repeated experiences or perceptive vividness.

2. DIAGNOSTIC METHODS

Diagnostic Clues

Children differ markedly with respect to symptoms, defenses, and level of ego organization within the same diagnostic category. The behavior of the same child is strikingly fluctuating; symptoms can sometimes be reversed, extended for periods of time, or even temporarily disappear depending on the age of the child, and particularly environmental influences.

Bradley (1947) suggested as criteria used for diagnosing schizophrenic children: (1) a generalized retraction of interests from the environment; (2) disturbances of thought manifested through blocking, symbolization, condensation, perseveration, incoherence, and diminution; (3) defect in emotional rapport; (4) rigidity and distortion of effect; (5) alterations of behavior with either an increase of motility, leading to incessant activity, or a diminution of motility, leading to complete immobility or bizarre behavior; (6) irritability when seclusiveness is disturbed, and sensitivity to comment and criticism.

Goldfarb (1945a, 1945b, 1956) singled out the following diagnostic criteria: (1) uncertainness about own identity, (2) confusion about time, space, and person, and (3) aberrant receptor behavior, characterized by extremes in activity and disuse of distance receptors such as touch, taste, and smell.

Bender suggested the following diagnostic signs (1953, 1959): (1) disturbance of motor coordination, such as lack of spontaneity, motor hyperactivity, dissociated movements, (2) disorientation in time and space, (3) excessive emotional sensitivity, (4) inability to control emotions, (5) severe anxiety, (6) uneven intellectual development, (7) extreme dependence on one adult, and (8) social withdrawal.

Bender (1953) suggested the following subdivisions of childhood schizophrenia: (1) The "pseudodefective" type, either retarded in maturation or regressed after an early normal development, inhibited, withdrawn, often apathetic and mute, sometimes tense, anxious, and fearful of new things. Children of this type have poor eating and sleeping habits, have poor resistance against illness, and display infantile motor habits. (2) The "pseudoneurotic" type with phobias and fears shows stereotyped movements or tics and compulsive activities. Their thought, speech, and sensory experiences are distorted; they are frequently irritated, with temper tantrums, panics, cryings, and hysterical laughter. (3) The "pseudopsychopathic" type who hates the world and acts out antisocial or delinquent behavior.

The autistic syndrome was distinguished by Kanner (1943). Most autistic children have originally been diagnosed as severely feeble-minded, and psychometric tests have often supported such a diagnosis. However, careful observations and examinations have shown that these autistic children are not mentally retarded. Autistic children lack the ability to relate themselves in the ordinary way to people and situations; they are most often seen with a placid smile, monotonously humming.

Another category, namely, symbiotic infantile schizophrenia was introduced by Mahler (1952). The symbiotic child "craves for bodily contact and seems to want to crawl into you, but he shrieks at such contact. On the other hand, their biting, kicking and squeezing is an expression of their craving to incorporate, unite with, possess, devour and retain the beloved. There is a fusion between the self and the mother, and a lack of direction between libidinal and aggressive tendencies . . . both the mother and the child are confused and fused as the goal of unneutralized instinctual forces" (Mahler, 1958).

Diagnostic Difficulties

Apparently, all the above-mentioned criteria for diagnosing schizophrenia in children are not specific enough. The broadness of these categories causes psychologists and psychiatrists to diagnose autistic and mentally deficient children as schizophrenic and schizophrenic children as mentally deficient.

Despert and Sherwin (1958) have tried to offer a diagnostic system that could help in distinguishing between schizophrenia, autism, and mental deficiency. They described three case histories stressing diagnostic clues as follows:

1. The first child described was destructive, experienced great fantasies and followed a rigid routine. After a period of psychological treatment, he was able to accept changes in his routine and began to speak. This child was diagnosed as schizophrenic.

2. The second child also had a rigid, patterned routine, was destructive, withdrawn, and failed to communicate. However, there was little improvement with treatment. This child did not smile and practiced a great deal of rocking while the first child did less rocking and more smiling. The second child was diagnosed as autistic.

3. The third child did not show early signs of speech impairment or rigid insistence on sameness of the environment. He was affectionate and able to relate to others, but disorganized in daily life. This child was given a strong anesthesia at the age of six months old and had become mentally defective.

According to Despert and Sherwin, impairment of communication is a symptom common to all three types of illnesses, but the extent of speech impairment is a useful diagnostic clue. The insistence on the sameness of the environment is another diagnostic clue characteristic of the autistic child. Mentally deficient children, however, are characterized by an over-all retardation in intellectual functioning and motor development.

It seems quite apparent that all these diagnostic clues lack precision. Several psychometric and projective techniques have been used by scores of research workers struggling with the problems of differential diagnosis. These problems are complicated by several factors, especially growth and interaction.

Diagnostic work with an adult patient assumes that unless the patient undergoes successful treatment, the diagnostic evaluation is valid. Diagnostic work with children cannot, however, claim the same validity, because of changes in their personality caused by the sheer process of growth and development. A five year old latent schizophrenic child may or may not become schizophrenic 10 years later. Prediction is not the most precise part of psychopathology, and it becomes even more difficult in regard to children because of the impact of growth and development.

Developmental processes depend largely on *social interaction,* especially in early years. Social interaction may considerably influence the child's performance on a diagnostic test. A review of schizophrenic responses on mental tests follows:

Garmezy (1952) shed additional light on this problem. He trained acute but cooperative schizophrenics and normal controls in auditory perception involving the ability to descriminate tones. In one test reward was given for a proper discrimination of tones; in another test reward was given for correct answers and a mild punishment administered for incorrect ones. In the first set of experiments there were but minor differences between acute schizophrenics and normals. When exposed to mild punishment, schizophrenics failed on the test and gave up efforts to improve.

A threat of failure may impair the intellectual functioning of schizophrenics. However, if the threat does not come directly from the supposedly friendly figure, be it a therapist, a parent, or an experimenter, but is an external threat, schizophrenics may work better (Wolman, 1957, 1958b). In an experiment conducted by Pascal et al. (1953), schizophrenics attained the same level of performance when exposed to a loud, threatening, and distracting noise. My interpretation is that an external threat helps to shift mental energies from the superego to the ego. When a threat comes from an emotionally neutral source such as inanimate nature, animals, or strangers, this threat forces a flow of energies into the protective apparatus, the ego. When the ego becomes libido cathected, the performance on the task improves.

The fact that motivation greatly influences the level of intellectual functioning of schizophrenics was demonstrated by Huston and Shakow (1946). Schizophrenic performance on motor learning was less efficient than the performance of normal controls. However, when an experimental group of schizophrenics was encouraged and prodded, their performance reached about the normal level.

Performance on a test depends largely on the attention of the experimental subject. Apparently most schizophrenics are overattentive to detail and underattentive to the over-all task.

Impairment of attention has been the subject of extensive studies in the U.S.S.R. Hamburg (in Russian, Gamburg) reported experiments with auditory stimuli and mild electric shock on 69 schizophrenics. Normal individuals respond with alertness, called by the Russians "orientation reaction," that is, increase in muscular and autonomic activity and electroencephalic frequency. Paranoid schizophrenics reacted defensively to the stimuli; simple schizophrenics did not react at all. While this behavior can be interpreted in terms of Pavlov's "protective inhibition" (see Malis, 1961), it can also be interpreted as an unconscious fear of doing anything that might be an invitation to criticism (Wolman, 1957, 1958b).

Schizophrenics are "children of mood"; in a happy mood, when they feel accepted—i.e., when they receive libido cathexes—they are at their best. When they feel rejected, specially by those whom they love or respect, their performance may go down. This is probably the reason why research workers cannot agree as to whether there is any substantial decline in mental functions in schizophrenia.

While over-all mental decline in schizophrenia can be doubted, peculiarities in the intellectual functioning of schizophrenics have been noticed. Piotrowski (1937, 1945) and other research workers noticed that schizophrenic children perceive on Rorschach minute details with great precision and then proceed to elaborate while overlooking larger details (see also Part 3, "The Rorschach Inkblot Method").

This overattention to detail is not necessarily a product of an impairment in cognitive processes; it may also represent a peculiar manner of relating oneself to the world. The tendency to hypercathect certain objects must lead to hypocathecting of others. A schizophrenic may become attached to a minute detail and overlook everything else. . . .

I am inclined to believe that the irrational thinking and acting of schizophrenics is produced to some extent by the *situation* in which the schizophrenic finds himself *here and now*. Schizophrenia is an escape into a lower level of functioning (downward adjustment). When the ego fails, some sort of morbid adjustment is made. Schizophrenia is a morbid way of living adopted when every other way seems to have failed (Wolman, 1965b, pp. 992-993).

Apparently, differential diagnosis of childhood schizophrenia is not an easy task. When schizophrenic children attain some level of intellectual development and acquire speech, they usually perform better on verbal than on nonverbal test items (Piotrowski, 1937, 1946). However, their over-all mental performance is uneven, largely depending on the areas of inhibition, often on their mood, attention, and relationship to the examiner. Mentally retarded children usually perform in an even and consistent way, but a schizophrenic child may fail on items he knows, and at a retest surprise the examiner. However, many pseudo-amentive and autistic schizophrenic infants do not respond to mental tests, nor do they react to the examiner. If and when they improve, their I.Q. keeps growing with the progress of treatment.

Perhaps the best summary of the problems encountered in diagnosing childhood schizophrenia was offered by Florence Halpern in Wolman's *Handbook of Clinical Psychology,* as follows:

. . . the *schizophrenic child* shows a variety of pictures, ranging from extreme autism to relatively mild yet characteristic schizophrenic departures from normal concepts and normal functioning. In other words, schizophrenia, like any other illness, can run the gamut from slight to very severe. Again as in the organic child, the severity will depend in part at least on the age at which the disturbance became manifest, the innate resources the child can mobilize in his adjustive efforts, and the attitude of the environment toward him and his illness. The common factors in all these cases, severe or mild, is the child's inability to perceive and experience himself in a stable, integrated fashion; to set firm ego boundaries;

and to come to terms with reality in an organized, meaningful fashion. Instead, because of the vague, fluid nature of his ego, he experiences both himself and his environment in a diffuse, disorganized manner. Lacking inner stability and organization, he cannot cope constructively with inner or outer pressures. In his case, the ego has erected no "protective barrier," and consequently he is being perpetually flooded by his own primitive, autistic needs and feelings. Correspondingly his reactions are frequently of a deviant, inappropriate, even bizarre order. At the mercy of his impulses, he can perceive the world only as a wild, confusing, dangerous, threatening place, and he reacts to it accordingly, defending himself against it either by withdrawing or by striking back against the objects that he thinks will destroy him. . . .

In the intellectual sphere, this highly uneven way of performing is often reflected in the extreme scatter that the subject shows on the intelligence test. For instance, on the Stanford-Binet a 7- or 8-year old child may base at year V and continue to have successes through XIV. Similarly, on the WISC, there may be as much as a 12-point or more difference between the low and high score that the schizophrenic child attains. Possibly even more typical for the schizophrenic is the unevenness that characterizes his functioning on any one subtest. He is very likely to fail some easy items, then pass more difficult ones, and continue in this fashion. There is no correlation between the difficulty of the task and his handling of it. Variable effort and attention at the time of testing, as well as very scattered, fragmented observations of the environment and what the environment offers him, seem largely responsible for this rather characteristic way of reacting. . . .

In addition to observation of the schizophrenic's behavior in the home, in school, on the playground, etc., personality testing can add a great deal to the understanding of the child's disturbance and his reaction to that disturbance. For example, the unstructured nature of the Rorschach can evoke highly disorganized reactions from the schizophrenic child who is constantly being overwhelmed by every kind of stimulus. In such cases all the indications of "primary-process behavior," lack of reality testing, primitivity, and confusion are rampant. The child simply uses the test stimulus as a springboard for his own highly idiosyncratic associations and makes no effort to bring these in line with more usual concepts. At such times the excessive concreteness and inadequate organizing and integrative abilities of the schizophrenic also become apparent. Thus he can give such interpretations as "A man with three legs and his tail is coming out of his nose and he has two eyes in his tail and he's coming right at me," etc. On the other hand, there are the schizophrenic children who are trying to make order out of inner and outer chaos and who do this by resorting to the commonly employed defenses, particularly withdrawal, denial, repression, blocking, and projection. The picture that emerges from such child's test protocol will then have many neuroticlike features, but despite all his attempts to adjust, his innate weaknesses will result in occasional breaks of a kind not seen in the neurotic or organic child. However, the fact that the child is trying to adjust, is using his assets in a reasonably positive fashion, certainly points to somewhat more positive utimate adjustment, provided the environment appreciates and supports his efforts, than is likely to be found in the case of the child who does not have enough resource or desire to make such efforts.

Just as the Rorschach serves as a kind of green light for a release of the child's autistic concepts, so too the CAT or TAT often produces a similar reaction. The child is very likely to start off his story in a way which indicates that he has recognized what the stimulus is, but he then proceeds to move away quickly from that stimulus, the child's initial perception and concept, and the end product. What is more, the child's productions are so confused, illogical, and irrelevant that it is often difficult, at times even impossible, to follow him. . . .

Very frequently, observation and "interview" with a schizophrenic child are sufficient to establish the diagnosis. However, intelligence testing not only substantiates the diagnostic impression but also gives a measure of the degree to which impairment is greatest. It likewise points out those areas in which he may be functioning in highly accelerated fashion, all of which can be useful in arranging an educational program for the child. Personality testing gives a picture of the way in which the child perceives himself and his world; how he is trying to meet the problems that every child, schizophrenic and nonschizophrenic, must face; and what his defensive operations are and where they can be strengthened and where they must be changed. For example, the schizophrenic child who, with the aid of obsessive-compulsive techniques, manages to stay in the environment and function with the same degree of effectiveness can be helped in these efforts, whereas the child who resorts only to denial and projection presents a very different picture in terms of educational planning and possible therapy. . . .

The number of personality pictures presented by the children in this group is astronomical. The common factor is the difficulty they have in adjusting to their world, inner and outer, and their inability to bring their own impulses and feelings in line with environmental expectations without feeling frustrated, anxious, or angry. To reduce these feelings and effect some adjustment, they resort to neurotic types of defense or act out their problems directly in their contacts with others. However, although their difficulties cause them to function less adequately than they otherwise might, in certain areas and under certain circumstances, and although they tend at times to be quite self-defeating, the deviations and distortions they manifest are not of a bizarre order and can generally be related dynamically to the child's life experiences. Just why the child chooses a particular form of adjustment or manifests a particular symptom seems in part to be a result of the specific nature of his disturbance and in part a result of the character of his environment. Many far more subtle factors have an impact on this matter of choice of symptom.

It is the function of the clinician to try to isolate and understand as many of these factors as possible, the better to appreciate what the symptom is communicating and thus acquire a better understanding of the child. . . .

The way the child perceives and reacts to the interviewing and/or testing situations sheds considerable light on his attitudes toward adults, especially those he perceives as authority figures, and also on the way he would like others to perceive him. Some of these children are made quite anxious by the experience, fearful that they may not perform as well as they think they are expected to or that they may say something they should not say, something that would not be acceptable. Hence they respond hesitantly and cautiously, and their very concern about themselves and the impression they are making tends to handicap them, to reduce their efficiency. These are the children who are dependent on the environment to the point where they will do almost anything to win environmental approval. Their efforts in this connection often take a considerable toll insofar as self-realization and the capacity for happiness are concerned. They are different from those children who constantly ask whether what they have done or what they have said is "right," "smart," "good," etc. Such children also want to impress others and surely have doubts about their adequacy and acceptability, but they are responding to their doubts with attention-getting, assertive forms of behavior, in contrast to the overly anxious, doubt-ridden reactions of the child who produces slowly and tentatively and who is obviously devoting all his effort and energy toward pleasing those about him who are important to him.

Some children reduce the concern the particular situation mobilizes by the adoption of an indifferent attitude. Anything that seems at all difficult to them, that requires any real effort on their part, is likely to be met with a shrug or an "I don't know." They allay whatever sense of discomfort their limitations might evoke by refusing to get involved, refusing to expose themselves to possible frustration or failure. Still other children go the opposite extreme, never admitting that any experience or any task is too much for them. Thus when a question on the intelligence test is well beyond them, they sit as if considering it, and nothing happens until the examiner suggests they try something else. When admission of failure is inevitable, they find justification for their shortcomings or put the blame for them onto the environment. Thus instead of "I don't know" they say "We didn't learn that yet," "My mother didn't tell me, "There aren't enough pieces so nobody could do it," etc. Then there are the talkers, the jokers, the laughers, who either are unconcerned or try to convince themselves and others that they are not troubled by the experience, even when it is obviously anxiety-evoking to them. . . .

Testing with this group of children serves many important functions. Because of the very important part that school and formal intellectual functioning play in the child's life, intelligence testing (unless of course there is a full, reliable report of recent testing available) should always be undertaken. Although the interest patterns obtained from this group of subjects will vary greatly and although differential diagnosis based on the findings of the intelligence scale is not as feasible as in the case of organic and schizophrenic children, the test results can indicate whether the child is being subjected to too much or too little pressure where intellectual achievement is concerned and whether his anxieties and his efforts at dealing with these anxieties are interfering somewhat with the effectiveness of his functioning. For example, the overly tense or pre-occupied child will have difficulty in concentrating and the rebellious child may show a marked inability to deal as adequately as he might with tasks requiring disciplined effort, such as arithmetical reasoning. . . .

The choice of projective tests depends, as it does in the adult, on what particular facets of the personality are to be explored, what particular problems need special investigation. The Rorschach is almost always indicated as the instrument best able to give a picture of pesonality structure and functioning, including the kinds of experiences that are most threatening to the child, the defensive techniques employed, and the effectiveness of these techniques. There are normative (Ames et al., 1952), and clinical (Halpern, 1953) studies dealing with the child's Rorschach responses at different age levels, normal and abnormal.

The CAT or TAT (Rabin and Haworth, 1960) fills in the picture obtained from the Rorschach, offering evidence of the way the child feels about many of his relationships and experiences and what he feels he can do about the distubances that these relationships and experiences produce. The Make-a-Picture-Story Test by Schneidman (1960) is a test that older children enjoy, and the fact that they have a free choice of characters and can bring into, and leave out of, the situation whomever they please has certain distinct advantages in evauating their ways of perceiving and structuring their experiences.

For most children, drawing a person is a much less upsetting kind of experience that it is for adults. The majority of children enjoy this task, and it often proves a good way of starting the testing session. It provides one way of evaluating the level of maturity that the child has obtained where his own body image is concerned. The 10-year-old who still produces little more than a round head set upon an egg-shaped body with no intervening neck and who indicates arms and legs simply by drawing sticklike projections from this egg-shaped body has a self-concept that is more in line with that of a 5-year-old child than a boy of his age. If his intellectual functioning is that of a 10-year-old, this disparity becomes all the more meaningful. Assessment of the drawing can be made by use of Goodenough's (1926) scoring technique and clinical evaluation (Hammer, 1958; Machover, 1949). In addition to a determination of the level of maturity reflected in the drawing, specific areas of disturbance often find expression in the emphasis or deemphasis of certain aspects of the figure. For instance, oral aggression is often revealed by a large mouth filled with enormous teeth, feelings of inadequacy by the absence of arms, and depression of the small size of the figure and its placement at the very bottom of the paper. Some investigators have noted that anxious children draw figures that are more rigid and more "mutilated" than less anxious children (Halpern, 1965, pp. 628-634).

3. THE SOCIODIAGNOSTIC TECHNIQUES

Lack of Clear Categories

Apparently there are no valid and reliable diagnostic methods and frequently the diagnostic categories change on reexamination. Psychometric tests and projective techniques may be mutually complementary, but even a combination of various techniques may not prove adequate.

There are objective diagnostic difficulties inherent in the nature of childhood schizophrenia. As mentioned above, schizophrenic behavior changes radically with the change of environment. No schizophrenic is always schizophrenic, and the nature and level of a schizophrenic's performance depends on how secure he feels. Schizophrenic children are even more fluctuating because they are children and in addition to the morbid schizophrenic process, the processes of growth and development affect behavior.

In addition to these diagnostic problems typical for childhood schizophrenia, a diagnostician faces almost insurmountable difficulties stemming from the lack of clearly established classificatory terms. If, for instance the term, autism includes both psychogenic and somatogenic disorders (Rimland, 1964), a differential diagnosis between organic and nonorganic disorders is rendered impossible.

Another difficulty stems from psychoanalytic interpretation of schizophrenia. Whether one agrees with Freud or with Federn (see Chapter 1), there is no doubt that schizophrenia represents a severe disorganization of the ego or lack of its development. However, the term "ego" does not convey any empirical data; it is a useful theoretical construct, and theoretical constructs evade empirical test.

Esman (1960) described some of the diagnostic difficulties. According to Esman, "doubts have arisen as to the utility of the term 'childhood schizophrenia,' and questions have been raised as to its precise clinical referents." Katan and Rank, among others, are against using the term "childhood schizophrenia." The best example given for not using this term is shown by Clardy and Rumpf (1954); of 32 children in Rockland State Hospital diagnosed as childhood schizophrenics, only nine retained that diagnosis after further study. "Other workers have experienced great difficulty in assigning such gradients as 'borderline,' 'schizoid personality,' and 'schizophrenia without phychosis' to specific child patients." What is being described in all cases is a state of severe ego disorganization or maldevelopment or both."

"The questions 'is this child schizophrenic or borderline?' or 'is this child who is not psychotic still schizophrenic?' do not arise when it is clear that the terms 'psychotic' and 'borderline' refer to gradients of ego disorganization rather than to specific psychopathological entities." There are children called "potential schizophrenics," which is really a misnomer because "ego disorganization" and "regression" are not the same as schizophrenia. Not even "transient states of ego disorganization under severe stress makes a child schizophrenic."

According to Beres, a clear picture "of the child's ego state and the various forces impinging on it" can be received through a careful outline of "those ego functions which are impaired and those which the more or less intact, together with a thorough assessment of the multiplicity of the possible etiological factors." There is no commitment to one "diagnostic entity with blurred outlines and controversial criteria." This also gives a good framework for "remedial or therapeutic efforts" without the black market connected with the diagnosis of "childhood schizophrenia." For we must remember that ". . . grave injustice is done to the child who is inaccurately diagnosed, since the diagnosis becomes a part of his life henceforth . . . [and] there is a certain degree of malignancy [associated] with the term 'schizophrenia'."

Classification

I do not have a remedy for all these and other diagnostic problems, but I believe that a reasonably consistent classificatory system may substantially reduce diagnostic difficulties.

An adequate classificatory system must fulfill at least two conditions, namely *economy* and *usefulness*. A classification is economical if no classified object belongs to more than one class and no object is left unclassified. The classificatory system of the American Psychiatric Association (1968) is open to criticism, because (1) after dividing all mental disorders into organic and nonorganic, it established a third category of mental deficiencies; (2) it forms a separate category of psychophysiologic disorders, while these disorders accompany a variety of other clinical categories such as, e.g., hysteria or schizophrenia.

Mental disorders can be classified in more than one way, but a scientific classification is useful when it *explains* the present situation by involving past *causes*. Certainly one can divide mental disorders according to symptoms, but a useful classification is based on *etiology*.

Moreover, a useful classification of mental disorders is one that is applicable to diagnosis, prognosis, and treatment. Such a classification must not use invisible and unobservable theoretical constructs such as ego, drive, etc. It must use observable behavioral clues.

Sociopsychosomatic Theory

The theoretical framework for the proposed classificatory system (briefly described in Chapter 1) was developed in a series of experimental studies in social psychology reported elsewhere (Wolman, 1956, 1958a, 1960, etc.) Those and other studies described human relation in three observable categories. Individuals relate to each other in terms of "receive" (get), "give and get," and "give" attitudes. The infant's attitude to mother is "to get"; his attitude is *instrumental,* for the mother is instrumental in satisfaction of his needs. Marriage is a "give and get" or *mutual acceptance* relationship. Parenthood is a "give" or *vectorial* type of relationship. Obviously, a well-adjusted individual participates in social relations on all three levels. Some of them (such as business) are instrumental; friendship and marriage are mutual; mature parenthood is vectorial.

Thus my main sociopsychosomatic hypothesis reads: *Whenever an organism (1) is exposed to adverse environmental conditions, (2) these conditions affect mental functions and personality structure and, consequently, (3) also affect the neurophysiological functions of the organism.*

Accordingly, the study of schizophrenia must include environment, personality, and organisms and be conducted by continued efforts of social psychology, psychology, and neurophysiology. This theory of mental disorders introduces a new classification of mental disorder, based on the psychological research of Freud, Federn, and others, on the neurophysiological research of Pavlov, Bykov, and others, and on the sociopsychological studies of Wolman.

The disturbance in the interindividual cathexes disrupts normal development and may cause permanent and severe disbalance in the self- and object-cathexes of both libido and destrudo. When in the formative years of childhood, love is not given to the child, the child's personality will develop in the direction of an extreme instrumentalism, as if resorting to the defensive-exploitative hostile attitude. *Hyperinstrumentalism* corresponds to what is usually called psychopathy, or sociopathy.

When the parental attitudes are inconsistent and the child is alternately loved and hated, protected and rejected, the child cannot develop an adequate give and take attitude. In this *dysmutuality* the inconsistecy of feelings is paramount. Love and hate for others come in cycles; love and hate for oneself, usually called elation and depression respectively are the most significant elements of this disorder, which in extreme cases is called the *manic-depressive* psychosis. Both object love and self-love are highly inconsistent.

If, however, parents demand love from the child instead of giving it to him, a peculiar disbalance is created. The child is forced too early to accept the extreme vectorial attitude and offer love and protection to his parents.

The lavish object hypercathexis prevents self-cathexis and causes a dangerous loss of own resources and decline in self-protection. Hypervectorialism leads to schizophrenia.

Classificatory System

Each of the three types of mental disorder can cause mild or severe mental impairment. There are five *levels* of this impairment: neurosis, character disorder, latent psychosis, manifest psychosis, and dementia (Wolman, 1965b). Not all patients go through all the five stages. Some start at a certain stage, and no significant deterioration takes place. Some start at a more severe level, for example, childhood psychosis. Some go through certain stages. But the five levels of stages represent the five potential degrees of deterioration in each type of disorder. (See Table 1.)

TABLE 1
Classification of Mental Disorders

Levels	Types		
	Hyper-instrumentalism, I	Dysmutualism, M	Hyper-vectorialism, V
Neurotic level	Hyperinstrumental neurosis (anxiety and depressive neuroses)	Dysmutual neurosis (dissociative and conversion neuroses)	Hypervectorial neurosis (obsessional, phobic, and neurasthenic neuroses)
Character neurotic level	Hyperinstrumental character neurosis (Sociopathic or psychopathic character)	Dysmutual character neurosis (cyclothymic and passive-aggressive character)	Hypervectorial character neurosis (schizoid and compulsive character)
Latent psychotic level	Latent hyperinstrumental psychosis (psychopathic latent psychosis)	Latent dysmutual psychosis (manic-depressive latent psychosis)	Latent vectoriasis praecox (latent schizophrenia)
Manifest psychotic level	Hyperinstrumental psychosis (psychotic psychopathy and moral insanity)	Dysmutual psychosis (manifest manic-depressive psychosis)	Vectoriasis praecox (manifest schizophrenia)
Dementive level	Collapse of personality structure		

Schizophrenia in childhood cannot be divided into clear-cut categories. Table 2 presents the various syndromes in order of increasing severity.

Observational Techniques

These syndromes are not mutually exclusive, and the same child may progress and regress, crossing the lines and even combining elements of several syndromes.

This fact makes one aware of the necessity of paying utmost attention to every *individual child* and, within the limits of broad

TABLE 2
Childhood Schizophrenia

Neurotic level (obsessive and phobic syndromes)	
Character neurotic level	
Latent psychotic level	
Manifest psychotic level	⎧ Aretic syndrome
	⎨ Symbiotic syndrome
	⎬ Autistic syndrome
	⎩ Pseudo-amentive syndrome

classificatory concepts, of assessing his particular potentialities. Several students of child psychopathology have developed highly specialized observational techniques.

One of the most frequently used methods of observing children is to observe them in *play* (Sorosky et al., 1968). Other means of observation include *visiting* the child in his home, thus studying his behavior in a natural environment, or observing the child in a nursery to watch the child in *social interaction.*

Other workers suggest a child-parent interaction study with the aid of tape recorders (Call, 1964). Some workers have observed children through a oneway mirror, narrating their behavior and changes in movement on a tape recorder. Through using proper observation procedures one is apt to obtain detailed information about the child which will suggest a treatment method most suitable for the particular child.

Sociopsychodiagnostics

In long years of work in hospitals, clinics, and private practice I have developed certain techniques to be described below. These techniques are far from perfection, and are offered as a proposal and suggestion for additional research. The advantage of these techniques lies chiefly in the fact that they (1) deal with *observable* phenomena of the individual's behavior, interaction, and communication with others, (2) are based on a systematic classification of the mental disorders, (3) are related to etiology and dynamics and not only to changing patterns and symptoms, and (4) may be of help in determining the strategy of therapeutic interaction.

The Sociopsychological-Diagnostic Inventory of Observation and the Sociopsychological-Diagnostic Interview roughly correspond to the techniques of statogram and self-statogram, respectively. In the Inventory of Observations, the observer or observers carefully record the overt patterns of behavior of the subject and categorize them in terms of power and acceptance. The observers register empirical data, record them carefully, and tabulate. To increase the objectivity of observations one can employ several observers, as reported in one experimental study (Wolman, 1956) and correlate their ratings. This observation includes actions (eating, sleeping, working, entertainment) and interaction and communication with other individuals.

The Sociopsychological-Diagnostic Interview reflects the subject's perception of himself and his environment in terms of power and acceptance. The interviewer conducts an open-end, focused-type interview (Merton and Kendall, 1964). The subject is requested to tell his life history, dwell on his childhood memories, describe his achievements and failures, describe his past experiences, etc. The interviewer avoids asking any direct questions; he encourages a free flow of communication and whenever necessary tries to bring out a point by asking questions such as "And what happened next? What have you done? How did you feel about it? And what was the reaction of others?" etc.

Hypervectorials display a great deal of *empathy,* i.e., they sense the feeling of others. Instrumentals have very little empathy, if any. Dysmutuals have less empathy than hypervectorials and more than hyperinstrumentals. Schizophrenics are not always friendly, but they are usually understanding; psychopaths do not care about others; manic-depressives go from one extreme to the other.

Hypervectorials excel also in *sympathy.* Hyperinstrumentals have no sympathy and no mercy, but they expect sympathy from others. Dysmutuals go to extremes; occasionally they are hypersympathetic and self-sacrificing and swing back to an almost psychopathic cruelty. Hypervectorials are cruel when furious; hyperinstrumentals are cruel when it pays to be; dysmutuals are cruel when agitated.

Hypervectorials in neurotic, latent psychotic, and remissive phases are usually *tactful* and *considerate;* they are often cold and cruel in schizo-type character neuroses and manifest schizophrenia. Psychopathic hyperinstrumentals are tactful toward those they perceive as strong and tactless and brutal toward those they perceive as weak.

Dysmutuals are oversentimental toward those whose love they wish to get and brutal toward those they do not care for; they are rarely tactful.

Moral rigidity characterizes hypervectorials; lack of morality is typical of hyperinstrumentals; moral inconsistency is the sign of dysmutuals. Hypervectorials cling to principles, are dogmatic and self-righteous. Hyperinstrumentals have no moral principles whatsoever; they are radical opportunists. Dysmutuals are highly idealistic and moralistic in one situation and the reverse in another. Hyperinstrumentals try very hard to be God-like angels and fear they are devils; when defenses fail, their destrudo erupts in a wild violence. Hyperinstrumentals are overtly selfish and unfair and believe they are within their rights. The whole world seems to be one *Lebensraum* for their ever-hungry wolf jaws, while they believe themselves to be innocent sheep. Dysmutuals are Dr. Jekyll and Mr. Hyde. When they feel rejected, they become brutal and aggressive.

Hypervectorials tend to *blame* themselves; hyperinstrumentals blame others; dysmutuals do both.

All disturbed individuals are prone to tell *lies*. Hyperinstrumentals lie whenever it is profitable. Hypervectorials rarely lie but may do so if their self-esteem is in jeopardy; they lie when they are afraid people will think they are bad or stupid. Dysmutuals lie frequently, usually for self-aggrandizement. Their lies are fantastic, often nonsensical; sometimes they say things that do not make sense even to themselves. Dysmutuals often sound insincere even when they are sincere.

The picture that hypervectorials have of other people is highly confused. They usually *perceive* others as better, stronger, smarter, than themselves and the members of their family. Their feeling of inferiority spreads to those for whom they feel responsible.

Hyperinstrumentals divide the world into those to fear and those to exploit. Dysmutuals divide the world into those who love and those who reject.

Hypervectorials are slow to form *friendships,* get lastingly overinvolved, and are unable to break off an attachment. Hyperinstrumentals have no friends on a give-and-take basis; a friend to them is someone to be exploited. Their friendships are formed for practical reasons and accordingly are either dropped or conveniently preserved. Dysmutuals easily develop profound attachments, but their feelings are rarely lasting.

Hypervectorials are most persistent and involved in *love.* When their love is not accepted, it turns into *hate.* Dysmutuals are never deeply in love, but they hate those who refuse to give love to them. Dysmutuals are "love addicts," constantly in search of new love objects. Their love is always ambivalent, and when it is not returned it becomes hate.

Sexual deviations accompany all mental *polymorphous perverts,* capable of and willing to participate in any type of sexual activity. Schizophrenics are frequently torn by the conflict of sex identification and fear of homosexuality. Manic-depressives frequently display impotence, frigidity, and other sexual disturbances.

The hypervectorials try to control hostility; they display *hostility* whenever rejected, offended, or unable to bear inner hostility, and when their defense mechanisms fail. Hyperinstrumentals are hostile whenever their needs are frustrated, that is, whenever their victims protest or anyone gets in their way. Their basic attitude is the defensive-aggressive hostility. The dysmutuals frequently show ambivalent hostility, hating friends who do not love them enough. A schizophrenic fights because he cannot control his hostile impulses; a psychopath fights to win; the manic-depressive vents his hostility whenever he is not loved. While hypervectorial schizophrenics are often hostile, they *cannot take hostility.* Blame or criticism sets off hostile reactions in hypervectorials. Hyperinstrumentals will accept criticism from those they perceive as strong and retaliate for criticism coming from weak individuals. Dysmutuals are not very sensitive to criticism coming from strangers but become aggressive-depressive (i.e., hostile toward others and themselves) when criticized by those who are expected to love.

The above-described behavioral differences must not be taken rigidly. As mentioned before, the environment, the age, and the particular individual traits must be always taken into consideration in diagnostic work.

CHAPTER 7

Psychotherapy

1. THE PSYCHOTHERAPIST

Vectorial Attitude

The main idea in psychotherapeutic interaction with latent and manifest schizophrenic children is to reverse the process of deterioration and to foster normal development. This therapeutic task is, perhaps, more complex and formidable than in adult schizophrenics. My assumption is that adult schizophrenics have experienced some degree of personality development; this development has been disturbed by hypervectorial interaction between the patient and his environment, and, at a certain point, regression has started. The aim of therapeutic interaction is, therefore, the restoration of an optimum of personality balance.

In childhood schizophrenia and especially in cases of infantile schizophrenia there has been very little, if any, personality development. The therapeutic task is therefore a dual one; on one hand, the noxious factors have to be counteracted; on the other hand, a re-education process must be started. The treatment of schizophrenic children is mainly "therapeutic education," or a combination of psychological methods of therapy with an over-all educational program aiming at the development toward normal adulthood.

The prognosis in childhood schizophrenics is believed to be the same as in adults. Most workers believe that "one third get better, one third fluctuate between better and worse, and one third get worse . . ." (Bender, 1968, p. 10). Eisenberg (1957) in a follow-up study was less optimistic and stated that only 25 per cent of schizophrenic children can be expected to attain a moderately good social adjustment during adolescence.

My own observations on this matter corroborate the opinion expressed in regard to the prognosis of adult schizophrenics (Wolman, 1966): *A schizophrenic becomes incurable when there is no one willing and able to cure him.* This statement must be emphatically repeated in regard to schizophrenic children.

Whatever has been said about the personality skills of the psychotherapist who works with schizophrenics has to be repeated in a magnified version in regard to therapists of schizophrenic children Unlimited willingness to give, true vectorialism, unswerving enthusiasm despite disappointments, never-ending patience in face of repeated challenges and provocations, and prolonged therapeutic cooperation with the not-always-cooperative parents are required in child psychotherapy.

The very fact that an adult person pays attention to the child whom nobody loved is in itself a powerful therapeutic factor. Thus, no matter what method has been used and irrespective of the therapist's theoretical premises, a friendly, giving, wittingly or unwittingly vectorial therapist may attain definite improvement. To quote Bender, all those who work closely with schizophrenic children "are convinced of a beneficial response to almost every method used" Bender, 1968, p. 10).

In the treatment of schizophrenic children, the personality of the therapist and the cooperation of the environment are the decisive factors in success, even to a greater extent than in the treatment of adults.

Psychotherapeutic Principles

The first principle is the principle of *graded reversal of deterioration,* a sort of "step-by-step-come-back" technique. When we work with a pseudo-amentive child, autism is a step forward; for an autistic child, the symbiotic syndrome is a step forward; aretic symptoms signify progress in a symbiotic child, and neurotic symptoms mean progress in any type of childhood schizophrenia.

We do not fight against symptoms, nor do we analyze them. An expression of disapproval of the child may cause additional withdrawal and further regression, and an analysis of syndromes may lay bare defenses. We do not remove, take apart, or take away whatever neurotic defenses the schizophrenic child possesses. *We build upon what we find.* If a child is symbiotic, we do not try to disrupt it, for a disrupted symbiosis will inevitably lead to autism or pseudo amentia. We build upon the symbiotic relation, support the symbiotic child and his mother until the symbiosis becomes unnecessary. One may compare this process to weaning; we do not take away the nipple but we offer a cup, and make the cup as attractive and satisfying as possible. The child will use both the cup and the nipple for a while, till he finds the cup so much more satisfying that he rejects the nipple.

This second principle is the principle of *constructive progress*. We do not take away anything; we add new, more mature, attractive, and tempting elements to the child's life. The schizophrenic child has stopped growing because growth seemed so dangerous; we must lure him, bribe him to grow and become adult.

The third principle is *education toward reality*. Psychotherapy with schizophrenic children, as with all schizophrenics, is primarily *ego therapy*. In regard to children, reality testing is the greatest problem. The child's temper tantrums, speech difficulties, inferiority feelings, his failures in controlling emotionality and mobility, and his lack of self-esteem must wait. As important as these symptoms are, they are second to reality testing. *Reality testing must receive top priority in the support of the failing ego in schizophrenic children.* The escape from reality in childhood is an escape from the social environment, and a refusal to grow and learn; it is an escape from life itself. The acquisition of factual knowledge is prevented and regression may take place to rock-bottom pseudo amentia. Therefore, working with schizophrenic children requires helping the child to get acquainted with the physical and social world, and shifting his attention from the inner world of fantasy and toward the real world of things and happenings.

Directive guidance is the fourth principle. This rule has to be explained in a broader context of the educational process. Education supports the natural process of growth from infancy to adulthood, but the term "adulthood" has different meanings in different cultures. To be "mature" has two connotations, biological and sociocultural. An adult is a biologically mature individual, irrespective of his society and culture. However, in accordance with its needs, society develops a set of culturally determined norms for adulthood and maturity. These norms are different in different times, cultures, and places. In ancient Greece "maturity" was different in Sparta and in Athens, and it is different altogether in our society today.

These sociocultural norms determine the cultural or *transcendent* goal of education according to the needs and norms of each society. The transcendent goal is the demand that children become well-adjusted adults in a *given* society. Thus education cannot be a laissez-faire system; its transcendent goal requires definite guidance, guidance towards the fulfillment of the sociocultural adjustment.

There is a similarity between education and psychotherapy. Education guides the individual development and learning toward normal adjustment in accordance with the imminent and transcendent educational goals. When this development and learning fail, corrective experience is necessary. This "emotional re-education" is the core of psychotherapy.

Obviously things went wrong with schizophrenic children. Since they are children, their psychotherapy cannot be merely a corrective emotional experience; it must encompass the totality of their educational experiences in the broadest sense of the word.

2. LEVELS OF TREATMENT

On the Lowest Level

Pseudo-amentive and autistic children are so afraid of human contact that even a highly skilled vectorial therapist must proceed with utmost caution. "The first requirement for treatment of the autistic child is to lure him into contact with a human love object. . . . Reactions which resemble parasitic-symbiotic mechanisms appear spontaneously or as an artefact of treatment. . . . The *autistic* child is most *intolerant of direct human contact.* Hence he must be lured out of his autistic shell with all kinds of devices such as music, rhythm activities, and pleasurable stimulation of his sense organs. Such children must be gradually approached with the help of inanimate objects, always keeping in mind that gross bodily contact, touching, cuddling—which one might expect would reassure a deeply disturbed child—is of no avail and often a deterrent with these autistic children. Time and again we see that causes of the autistic type, if forced too rapidly into social contact and into facing the demands of the social environment, are thrown into a catatonic state and then into as fulminant a psychotic process as we see in some of the symbiotic child psychoses" (Mahler, 1952, p. 301-

302). Similar observations have been reported by other workers (Bettelheim, 1950, 1955; Betz, 1947; and many others).

There are no clearly defined techniques as to how to approach a pseudo-dementive or autistic child. A prerequisite of success is an unconditional, accepting, vectorial giving attitude, but, as Bettelheim put it, "love is not enough." Severely disturbed schizophrenic children fear and distrust people because their parents acted and talked as if they were loving while they exploited the child emotionally. The "double-bind" (Bateson et al., 1956) is the prevalent communication pattern in all schizophrenic families. To convince the frightened little schizophrenic that this time this grown-up (the doctor) means what he says and does, and is really willing to help and not to exploit, requires special talent and skill. Psychotherapy with schizophrenic children is more than a technique to be learned; *it is an art based on scientific principles.* The scientific foundation of the therapeutic interaction must be studied thoroughly, but the day-by-day interaction with a highly disturbed and exceedingly sensitive little schizophrenic involves an application of scientific principles that requires talent and mastery.

I have seen therapists who displayed this mastery. There have been considerable differences in their personalities, philosophies, and training, but there have also been some definite personality and behavioral traits shared by all of them. All of them approached the withdrawn child without hesitation, as if not being able to talk was the most natural thing in the world for a four year old child, or as if banging the head or sitting for hours in a rocking chair was the right kind of leisure time. Their approach to the child was kind but not sentimental.

All successful therapists I have watched approached the child in a *matter-of-fact fashion.* They did not ask unnecessary questions, nor did they show any hesitation. Perhaps they felt intuitively or empathically what was the right thing to do. I have seen a psychiatric nurse go over to a screaming five year old boy and say, "Come on." She stretched out her hand and went with him for a little walk. The child accepted the hand, calmed down, and followed the lead. Two minutes later she offered him a cookie, which he took. The little scene took place after 30 minutes of desperate effort on the part of another nurse who argued against head banging, used bribes and threats, and got nowhere with the youngster.

Perhaps the child sensed that the first nurse was anxious, insecure, worried about his screaming, afraid that the child might hurt
himself, and anticipated criticism from the ward psychiatrist. In my
observations on hospital wards I noticed the impact of the staff
meetings on the staff-patient interaction and on the behavior of
schizophrenic patients. Being exceedingly sensitive, schizophrenics
are the first to notice tension and insecurity in the hospital staff and
react with their own increased tension (Wolman, 1964).

The second nurse who took the child for a walk was an elderly
woman, greatly respected and generally liked in the hospital, not
afraid to admit her errors. She was perhaps more involved with her
task but less involved with the patients and less misled by her own
countertransference feelings. There was little if any difference in
the overt actions or words of the two psychiatric nurses. Both
were friendly, both soft-spoken, both said, "Come on, Tommy," and
both stretched out a hand. It would be difficult to trace the success
of the second nurse to superior technique or skill. The difference
was in their personalities, in the emotional climate emanating from
them, and in the difference in their self-esteem. In psychotherapy
with both adults and children *being is far more important than doing
and personality is far more important than technique.*

Successful psychotherapists, such as J. L. Despert, E. R. Geleerd,
M. S. Mahler, B. Rank, and many others differ in details of technique, but all of them give the child the feeling of being uncondi-
tionally accepted, cared for, loved, and respected. All of them
appeared to the child as people who know what they want, self-
assured, strong, friendly, and infinitely patient. Whether they interpret the child's communications, verbal and nonverbal, via
Freud's or Sullivan's terminology, seems to be of secondary importance. What they *do* with the child, whether he is five or 10
years old, is to encourage his growth, to help him to perceive things
as they are, and to make him feel accepted and protected.

On the Symbiotic Level

Some children start on the autistic level and progress to the symbiotic level; some start on the symbiotic level and regress. The principle of graded reversal of deterioration must be applied with utmost caution in psychotherapy with children. As Mahler says (1952,
pp. 302-303):

In the *symbiotic type* . . . it is important to *let the child test reality very gradually at his own pace.* As he cautiously begins this testing of himself as a separate entity, he constantly needs to feel the support of an understanding adult, preferably the mother or the therapist as mother substitute. Such continual infusions of borrowed ego strength may have to be continued for a lifetime. In other words, *separation as an individual entity can be promoted only very cautiously* in the case of the symbiotic psychotic child. . . .

Prognosis as to arrest of the process and as to consolidation of the ego is moderately favorable. It seems to depend on the right type, and the cautious, prolonged, and consistent nature of the therapy, which is a kind of substitution of infusion therapy. However, the outlook as to real cure is bleak. . . .

Any pressure in the direction of sudden separate functioning must be cautiously avoided in the *symbiotic child.* If the ego of the symbiotic type is overrated and expected to be able to cope with reality without continual ego infusion from the therapist who substitutes for mother, the panic reactions and acute hallucinations may cause regressions and withdrawal into stuporously autistic states or hebephrenic deterioration. Therefore simultaneous supportive treatment of the mother, if at all possible, seems to constitute the optimal and, perhaps, even a *sine qua non* approach to the problem.

My experience has shown that any effort to insert a wedge between child and mother may lead to a catastrophic deterioration. The therapist, being fully aware of the damage inflicted on the child by his mother, must not express his feelings and opinions in this matter. The child already has ambivalent feelings toward his mother. When his ego has become sufficiently strong, perhaps the true nature of his mother's symbiotic needs can be cautiously explained, but the timing of the dissolution of this tie is of the greatest importance. A complete cure cannot be obtained without dissolution of symbiotic relations, but it has to come gradually, and not through psychoanalytic interpretation but through a support of the child's ego that will eventually make the symbiosis superfluous. Apparently, in some cases this may not be possible at all. Since too early a separation may lead to a catastrophy, the therapist should rather leave the initiative to the child. When the child becomes more outgoing, more self-assured, and more independent, he himself will reject his mother's overprotective attitude. However, even in such a case, the therapist should not too eagerly accept the child's lead; he must *not* join the little patient in condemnation of his mother. The eagerness of the therapist may be interpreted by the child as an accusation of the mother and an approval of the child's hostility towards her, and it may therefore elicit a profound guilt feeling or a storm of anxiety.

My own policy has been usually one of "buffering." While approving the young patient's striving toward independence, I have usually pointed out his mother's good intentions. It has always had a beneficial effect on the patient; it tempers his angry criticism of his mother and prevents, or at least alleviates, his guilt feelings. The image of a "bad mother" stirs in the child an uncontrollable desire to hurt and to destroy himself and others. While the therapist should never deny facts, he must not encourage hate and must not join in condemnation, but use soothing words and judgment in moderating. The therapist's joining the child against his mother is usually a countertransference phenomenon (Ekstein, 1953).

A similar problem often arises in the treatment of adult schizophrenics. There has been always a conflict in their minds concerning the role their mother has played in their life. As mentioned before, there is no real cure without severing this object hypercathexis (Wolman, 1966), but this severance is not always advisable or possible. In the case of an "overstayed childhood schizophrenic," any effort to break this bond may be dangerous. Some patients, much improved and otherwise well adjusted, may not be able to assume full independence, and thus remain attached to their mothers. In each single case the therapist must weight the pro's and con's of pressing or abandoning this issue. Pragmatic flexibility and strategic valuation of the patient's personality must be applied in each case. In the treatment of childhood schizophrenia, *individualization* and *flexibility* count among the greatest virtues. Psychotherapy with schizophrenic children is primarily a vectorial process of cathexis coming from the therapist. Or, in Mahler's words, it is sort of "infusion." An infusion cannot proceed blindly; it must take into account the personalities of both the giver and the receiver.

Therapeutic Interaction

The schizophrenic syndromes in childhood easily change and shift, interlock and overlap, and preschool and school-age children display a great variety of behavioral patterns. Geleerd's cases, for instance, displayed impulsive behavior; in group situations they are either "uncontrollably aggressive or completely withdrawn," in contrast to their "charm and wit when alone and undisturbed with one adult." They could not take frustration; they could not control their aggressive behavior as normal children did, nor could they respond well to firm handling as neurotic children did. A schizophrenic child "becomes more paranoid when treated with firmness. He considers it proof of his paranoid ideas. But a loving, soothing attitude of a familiar, affectionate adult will bring him back to normal behavior" (Geleerd, 1946, p. 272).

Hostility elicits hostility. Since hostility is, basically, a protective reaction of the organism to danger, hostility from without elicits hostility reaction in the organism. No one likes those who hurt, but a normal child may feel hostile to parents and teachers without acting out and without too much guilt feeling.

The problem of hostility is a crucial problem in psychotherapy with schizophrenic children. A genuinely friendly, affectionate, patient, vectorial adult may produce miraculous changes in a disturbed child. An impatient, irritable, overdemanding, punitive adult forces the child to regress to a lower level of adjustment in accordance with the principle of downward adjustment in schizophrenia.

Schizophrenic children are referred for treatment mostly because of their destructive behavior. The aretic syndrome is probably the most frequent one, but other types are also easily aroused and destructive. Unlimited permissiveness of the therapist provokes anxiety, and anxiety may turn into vehement hostility. So does the therapist's restrictive firmness; it provokes a senseless fight for independence almost resembling the fight for survival. Obviously there is no other therapy but "protective love" offered by an understanding, firm, and absolutely reliable adult. This is probably the secret of successful psychotherapy, but there are no definite general rules as how to practice it. As one child psychotherapist whom I supervised said, partly in despair, partly in jest, "You want me to be not too meek, not too strong; not too permissive, not too strict; not too close, not too distant; not too fast, not too slow; not too sympathetic, not too cold; not too lenient and not too domineering. Could you, at least, tell me just *how* to act in this particular case?"

There is no uniform and general answer to this question. The most general answer would be, "Act as a prudent and loving parent would. Would you threaten or punish a frightened child? Would you let him demolish your furniture, hurt himself and others?"

The schizophrenic child puts the therapist to a difficult test. He tries to annoy the therapist, to tease and provoke, and to find out whether the therapist will blame him as his mother did or beat him as the father did. The schizophrenic child senses the mood of the therapist and often misinterprets him. Whenever the therapist is tired or worried, the child thinks, "It is because of me. I am a bad child and even the doctor hates me." On the other hand, the child's hostility is not always a test; it is often an uncontrollable hostile impulse, an outburst of destrudo in an organism whose libido has been given away. It may be the "panic" or "terror" type of hostility; it may also be resentment. "Why aren't you my mother? Why must you be nice and my mother mean?" cried a 10 year old boy.

Disapproval of child's aggressive behavior helps the child to develop reality testing. The child begins to learn that there are adults who are friendly and do not get infuriated any time he does not do what they want him to do. They are not hostile, but they set firm limits.

Good psychotherapists think straight and are not masochistic; they are rational and know what is right and what is wrong; they convey to the child the message that he is not the omnipotent "bad guy," but that he must respect the rights of other people. If the child cannot control the impulses that frighten him so much, he may rest assured that the therapist will control him and help him to control himself.

The parents of schizophrenic children are rarely consistent. While they are usually critical of the child, the father being competitive and the mother demanding, both of them, being instrumental, actually depend on the child for emotional support, and both of them crave the child's love.

Being so dependent, they do not exercise parental authority. When they forbid a certain way of playing, it is not because the rational thing to do is to forbid a dangerous or improper way of playing but because it annoys them. When they allow it, it is not because it is right, but because they want to please or because they give up.

The therapist may be inclined in a countertransference to identify with the poor child, resent the bad mother, and become overpermissive (cf. Ekstein, 1953). When frustrated in his therapeutic efforts, he may resent the child's ungratefulness and lack of progress as the mother did.

It is, therefore, important to stay clear of countertransference involvement that may wreck any psychotherapeutic relationship. The psychotherapist must be what the child's parents never were, namely, a *rational adult*. He does not put the blame on the child, nor does he expect the impossible. He does not threaten, punish, or blame, but he does not yield to the child's irrationality.

When the child, driven by panic or rage, is actually out of contact with reality, reasoning will not help. Yet the therapist must not allow the child to hurt himself or others or destroy property. He must stop destructiveness, preferably by a soothing, affectionate attitude. The more one feels loved and protected, the less need there is to fight against true or imaginary enemies. Sometimes the child can be distracted, gotten interested in a toy, a tool, or a game. When one nerve center is stimulated and excited, the other centers become inhibited (Pavlov, 1928, p. 324 ff.). Sometimes there is no other way but physical restraint, gentle, friendly, yet firm.

Each time the therapist counteracts the child's destructive acting out in a friendly and firm manner without blaming the child and without interpretation, the child becomes less and less afraid of his own hostile impulses. But this is only a secondary task in psychotherapy. It is far more important to *prevent* hostile acts than to stop them. The total psychotherapeutic interaction is geared toward the increase of self-cathexis and self-esteem and improved ego control of impulses. A child who loves himself and feels loved is not destructive any more.

Interpretation and Insight

Here we come to the problem of interpretation and insight. Even orthodox analysts have expressed doubts as to whether treatment of schizophrenia should follow the pattern of classic psychoanalysis. Men like Bak (1954), Brody and Redlich (1952), Bychowski (1952), Eissler (1952), Federn (1952), Knight (1953), and many others have deviated from the method of free association and interpretation of unconscious phenomena. The prevailing opinion is that while in neurosis the repressed material has to be brought up to the surface by free association and interpreted, in psychosis repression of the unconscious may be the advisable procedure.

Even in manifest psychosis, where the conscious seems to be flooded anyway by the unconscious, one may doubt the wisdom of interpretation that may increase the flood. My policy has been to delay interpretations until adequate ego compensation symptoms have been established, and never to interpret when interpretation seemed to lay the defenses bare.

A schizophrenic child has little ego to fall back on, and interpretation does not seem to be of much help. Since the danger of harm is definitely greater than in adults, avoidance of interpretation is recommended in most cases. However, in a case of a mild teen-age patient, interpretation of two dreams has been of some value. The girl dreamt that a little fish bit and ate a big crab. Her immediate association was that her little brother had eaten and destroyed mother's breast and the mother might die. In the second dream a little cat was eating a big cat's liver. The girl associated herself with the little kitten and her mother with the big cat. Her mother's favorite expression was that her children have caused her liver disease.

The girl expressed profound guilt feeling. She blamed herself and her little brother for causing mother's sickness and eventually death. Analysis of the dreams helped to alleviate the guilt and present mother's disease in a realistic way.

Realistic perception of things and events is of crucial importance in psychotherapy with children. Children as a rule do not hallucinate, but they easily escape into the world of daydreaming and fantasies of omnipotence. The therapist must tactfully and constantly bring them back to the world of things as they are. The therapist must encourage (in and outside the therapeutic hours) interests and activities typical for children of the patient's age or as close to his age level as possible.

I see little advantage in the therapist's joining the child in a regressive journey. I doubt the therapeutic wisdom of permitting the child to neglect bowel control or smear feces or destroy things. The therapist, being an adult, must always represent the reality principle. The child's parents have acted as irrational adults. The therapist, acting as a rational adult, must start at the highest possible level of adjustment and foster the process of growth and learning.

Reality, always reality, is the keynote in psychotherapy. Realistic perception counteracts morbid megalomanias and inferiority feelings. The therapist should not spare encouragement; he may help the child to be successful in work and play and praise true achievements, but he must never abandon truth and reality.

Working with Families

One may doubt the possibility of successful psychotherapy with children without parental cooperation. The chances of helping a child against his parents' wishes are slim, but to assure parental cooperation is not an easy task either (cf. Peck et al., 1949). In practically all cases, the parents feel responsible for the child's illness and are overwhelmed with shame, anxiety, and guilt. Even if they themselves are not pathologic (in my sample about 50 per cent are), the schizophrenic child evokes hostility. The schizophrenic child is constantly hurt by his parents and constantly hurts them. Being over-involved with his parents, he is exceedingly sensitive to their moods and often interprets signs of fatigue or irritation caused by business disappointments, indigestion, or toothache as signs of parental rejection, or as signals of their approaching death. Slight and insignificant changes in parental moods elicit in the schizophrenic child feelings of helpless anger, directed towards himself and others.

The overt behavior of a schizophrenic child is often a challenge even to patient and understanding individuals. Parents of schizophrenic children, whether mentally disturbed or not, are disturbed in their interindividual relations. They are instrumental-exploitative to one another and toward the child. Frustration in instrumental relations easily turns into agitated hostile feelings. These feelings in the parents elicit additional tension in the child, and this in turn makes the parents even more hostile.

This vicious cycle may wreck the best psychotherapeutic work. Often the parents would like to cooperate and try very hard to be friendly and understanding. Yet when exposed to their child's actions, they quickly lose patience and soon become involved in a tug-of-war accusing each other for failing in the upbringing of the child. The mutual accusation leads to a flare-up and, even if the parents know they should spare the child, they cannot help using the child as a battlefield.

Parental discord and clashes drive the child to despair. The father, instead of being the leader and protector of the family, is a quarrelsome yet a spineless creature, competitive-seductive toward the child. The mother, instead of being the source of food and comfort, is the most threatening enemy. The schizophrenic child usually takes the side of the stronger party, but he lives under a frightening threat of losing one or both parents.

Then he begins to "protect" them. He controls the household by using bad language, banging his head, screaming, and violence. The frightened parents often yield to the child's terror and irrational demands. The child does not accept the reality principle, and does not learn to give up his whims and momentary needs for the future ones. He does not learn to accept the inevitable discipline and restraint and consideration for other people.

Unless the parents change the intrafamilial patterns of interaction, there is not much hope for successful psychotherapy with the child. I would therefore say that the participation of the parents in psychotherapy is a *conditio sine qua non* in psychotherapy with schizophrenic children. On a few occasions, in fact, I have seen the child at irregular intervals, while intensive psychotherapeutic work has been conducted with both parents. The results have been quite satisfactory.

In working with parents of schizophrenic children, whether it is guidance, psychotherapy, or group therapy, one must account for a great deal of unconscious resistance and conscious evasion. "I am sick and tired of listening to the psychiatrists who put all the blame on mothers," stated a mother of two schizophrenic children angrily. "Everybody blames me; my husband, the teacher, the school psychologist, the neighbors. The only thing I know is that my husband's brother is also mentally sick," said another mother.

The therapist who works with parents must avoid identifying himself with the child and blaming the parents. He *must not* make the parents feel guilty and perceive themselves as failures; such an attitude can adversely affect the intrafamilial relations. The therapist must gain a clear insight into the factors perculiar to each family and treat the parents of schizophrenic children at least with the same degree of objectivity and sympathy as a physician would treat the parents of a child with polio even if he suspected parental negligence.

A respectful, friendly, and sympathetic attitude may win over the parents and enable the therapist to make them understand the severity of the problem and the importance of interindividual relations. It is a serious mistake to work with the mother alone; such a situation, in which mother, child, and therapist form a triad with the exclusion of the patient's father, may create additional intrafamilial alienation and increase the schizogenic pattern of interaction. In fact, the father must play the decisive role in family psychotherapy and it seems advisable to start with the father. In most cases he is the least anxious family member because he is unaware of how guilty he is in the family drama. If the father changes his attitude and becomes a friendly husband and protective father, more than half of the task has been accomplished. The mother, pressured no more by her husband, may ease off her pressure and her emotional demands on the child.

It seems to be advisable to work with both parents together or at least simultaneously. Whether this work is guidance, brief psychotherapy, or deep psychoanalytic therapy varies from case to case.

There are no rules for adequate parenthood, but I would make the following eight suggestions to the parents:

1. Avoid conflict with the child. Remember, each tantrum is a step down.

2. Do not punish the child; do not use threats of abandonment nor physical violence. Punishment makes the schizophrenic child worse.

3. When the child is aggressive, distract him or disarm him by your friendly and soothing attitude. Overlook minor transgressions and stop major ones without getting hostile.

4. Offer positive guidance. Child education is not a laissez-faire experience, but a system of rational rules. Establish rules concerning table manners, bedtime, schoolwork, etc., and be consistent.

5. Be friendly but not overbearing, reliable but not domineering, offer help but do not overprotect. Allow the child to use his own initiative. Trust and encourage him whenever he tries new activities.

6. Stick to reality. Do not psychoanalyze your child. Do not criticize fantasy, but offer knowledge, facts, and skills.

7. Never talk about the child or your marital problems in the child's presence.

8. When father and mother become friendly husband and wife, the child's condition improves.

Several workers have pointed out the need of simultaneous parent-child psychotherapy. Sabbath (1955) described a mother who identified her child with her own invalid father and regarded all men, inclusive of her own husband, as injured (catastrated) people "whom she has to *take care* of and at the same time dominate." This mother, who punished the child for her own "bad" impulses, was preventing the child's treatment.

Kanner and Eisenberg reported a case of a four year old autistic and mute boy. The emphasis in therapy was put on the child's mother; the "newly established symbiotic relationship between her and the child brought about a marked improvement in the child" (Kanner and Eisenberg, 1955, p. 235).

There have been many similar cases reported in the last decade. There is, obviously, a growing awareness of the fact that schizophrenia is the product of weird family relationships, and that to cure schizophrenia one must improve family relationships (cf. Bowen, 1960; Jackson and Weakland, 1961; Midelfort, 1957; Peck et al., 1949; and others).

3. EDUCATIONAL PROBLEMS

The School

Intellectual regression is one of the worst prognostic signs, and it must be counteracted by all means. The schizophrenic child must be helped and encouraged to learn and acquire as much skill and knowledge as his intellectual capacities permit.

Which school for these children?

The answer is *as close to normal as possible*. The majority of schizophrenic children are best off in regular school with usual teachers and standard curriculum. Most schizophrenic children are capabale of doing the customary scholastic work provided they receive adequate attention, more encouragement, and more supervision than other children do.

Cooperation between the psychotherapist and the child's teacher is of paramount importance. Intelligent and conscientious teachers may accept the difficult child as a challenge; they may discover that in most cases their efforts are rewarded by the child's progress. Several teachers with whom I worked reported miraculous changes. The schizophrenic child's span of attention is short, and his thoughts often wander away from the work to his poor mother; he needs to be reminded, prodded, supervised, and encouraged to go back to reality. The school, the teacher, and objective knowledge may become important vehicles in the child's recovery.

A schizophrenic child can be helped to become *constructive*. It is of great therapeutic importance to encourage him and to help him to do well on a task, to attain real accomplishments, and to acquire factual knowledge and practical skills. Schoolwork brings the child closer to reality and makes him do what other children do. Every single achievement increases his self-esteem, makes life more attractive to him, and gives him courage to grow.

The relationship with other children represents a serious problem. The way to socialization leads through parental support and, in school, through the support of the teacher. Children are often cruel, but a good teacher may tactfully and discretely change the classroom atmosphere. Pushing a shy child and forcing him into group activity does not help. There seems to be a widespread belief that the schizophrenic child has to be coerced into participating in social life and made to spend maximum time with other children. Unfortunately, such a method never brings about the expected results. When a schizophrenic child who has failed to make friends in his neighborhood is sent away from home to a camp or to an institution, his feelings of loneliness and rejection increase and, most likely, he will become more withdrawn and more schizophrenic. On the other hand, the improvement of the intrafamilial interrelationship makes the child less schizophrenic and gives him courage in relating to other children.

What the child really needs is a *vectorial environment* in which love and affection will be given to him. In all my experience with psychotic children I have been most successful in those cases when parents or parental substitutes and teachers gave the child unconditional, affectionate support. Once the child's interindividual libido cathexes became better balanced and he felt loved and cared for without strings attached, his intraindividual, self-directed cathexes of libido became better balanced. The loved child begins to respect himself, becomes more self-assured, and exercises better self-control. Then, and only then, may be become capable of developing social relations on a mutual acceptance, give and take level.

Obsessional and phobic children and milder cases of childhood schizophrenia can benefit by a regular school provided the teacher can give them a little extra attention. The teacher cannot "cure" the child, but close cooperation between the therapist, the parents, and the teacher may prove exceedingly beneficial for the child.

Very severe cases from very disturbed homes need special education and institutionalization.

Remarks on Institutionalization

I have been always opposed to the removal of the child from his natural home environment. I believe that the disturbed child needs a home and parents and normal condition for growth and development. For many years I was director of a children's clinic and later supervisor of a network of clinics, and I did whatever I could to prevent institutionalization of children. If a child needs help, the help must be given to him while he lives in his home, and the help must be extended to his parents also.

Sometimes immature, selfish, instrumental parents want to get rid of the burdensome child and send him away to an institution, often wishing that he may never come back. In such cases, therapeutic efforts must be concentrated on the parents to help them to accept themselves and to accept their child. In most cases to take away the schizophrenic child from his home means to take him away from traumatic experiences and to push him into catastrophe. "Children who had been emotionally deprived (usually by institutionalization) in the first several years showed personality damage beyond repair" (Bender, 1956, p. 504).

Unfortunately, there are cases when institutionalization becomes inevitable because the child has no home or the home situation is desperately hopeless. Once I worked with a tragic case where a mother had tried to kill her three children and was hospitalized and the father had assumed full responsibility. The oldest boy was big enough to help; a psychiatric social worker took care of the family as a unit, and the family was preserved till mother came back home after being hospitalized for five years. Fortunately, the family bond was somehow preserved and the mother had a place to come back to. In another case the father was a drunkard who tortured the schizophrenic child, and the mother was a simple deterioration schizophrenic who did not care. There was no other way but to send the child away. In still another case the mother left, the father was gone, and the children were practically orphans with no one to care for them. Institutionalization may become inevitable when there is no one to take care of the child. Perhaps a foster home would be a better solution than an institution whenever it is possible to find good-natured, friendly, and sensible people willing to care for a child whose behavior is unbearable, who hates everyone and mostly himself, and who requires infinite love, patience, and understanding. Kanner (1949, p. 716) reported substantial improvement in a boy who went to live with an understanding and friendly aunt, was enrolled in a school where he was not pushed, and where he found a quiet, nonaggressive boy in whose company he felt increasingly comfortable. I have had the chance to observe a few cases of successful placement.

Some institutions are bad, and some are good, depending on the quality of the work and quantity of workers. Even the best counselors, therapists, and nursing and educational personnel may fail in an understaffed institution. Each schizophrenic child represents an enormous demand on human patience and on human resources, as Bettelheim's vivid descriptions prove (Bettelheim, 1950, 1955, 1967).

There have been several experimental approaches to family treatment.

According to Bettelheim, working with the mother and the child together is usually unsuccessful, and *treatment of a child who lives at home is extremely inefficient and often futile.* It is the presence, night and day, day in and day out, of a therapist who, in Anna Freud's words, "offers herself in the flesh . . . as a strong, ever-present object so that the patient's personality could be unified around this image. . . ." Bettelheim believes that schizophrenic children must be placed in surroundings outside the home. Once in this environment the child and his problems can be given full attention, and the child is helped independently of his mother. For each child the course of therapy is different.

The issue is controversial, and there have been several attempts to treat schizophrenic children in special schools, care centers, closed institutions, and hospital wards. The reader is referred to the excellent work of Bettelheim (1950, 1955, 1967), Redl and Wineman (1960), and other books and papers. The only remarks to be made here is that the impression gained from the reading of this material is that therapeutic success depends largely upon the ability of the workers to be vectorial and their opportunities to do so. Overcrowded and understaffed institutions with an impersonal attitude towards the child cannot claim much therapeutic success.

Apparently, there is more than one way of helping the schizophrenic child. The present chapter has outlined a tentative course of action without claiming that this is the only or the best method.

References

Abraham, K. *Selected papers on psychoanalysis.* New York: Basic Books, 1955.

Agras, S. The relationship of school phobia to childhood depression. *American Journal of Psychiatry,* 1959, *116,* 533-536.

Alanen, Y.O. The mothers of schizophrenic patients. *Acta Psychiatrica et Neurologica Scandinavia,* 1958, *33,* Supp. 724.

Alexander, F., and Flagg, G.W. The psychosomatic approach. In B.B. Wolman (Ed.). *Handbook of clinical psychology.* New York: McGraw-Hill, 1965, 855-947.

Altshuler, K.Z. Genetic elements in schizophrenia: A review of the literature and résumé of unsolved problems. *Eugenics Quarterly,* 1957, *4,* 92-98.

American Psychiatric Association. *Diagnostic and statistical manual of mental disorders.* Washington, D.C.: Author, 1968.

Ames, L.G., Learned, J., Metraux, R.W., and Walker, R.N. *Childhood Rorschach responses: Developmental trends from two to ten years.* New York: Hoeber-Harper, 1952.

Anderson, C. Organic factors predisposing to schizophrenia. *Nervous Child,* 1952, *10,* 36-42.

Aprison, M.H., and Drew, A.L. N₁N-Dimethyl phenylenediamine oxidation by serum from schizophrenic children. *Science,* 1958, *127,* 57-58.

Arieti, S. *Interpretation of schizophrenia.* New York: Bruner, 1955.

Bak, R. C. The schizophrenic defense against aggression. *International Journal of Psycho-analysis,* 1954, *35,* 129.

Bakwin, H. Emotional deprivation in infants. *Journal of Pediatrics,* 1949, *35,* 512-521.

Bakwin, H., and Bakwin, R. *Clinical management of behavior disorders in children.* Philadelphia: Saunders, 1960.

Baldwin, A.L. *Behavior and development in childhood.* New York: Dryden, 1955.

Baltrusch, H.G. Psychophysiologische Analyse einiger Funktionen der höheren Nerven Tätigkeit. *Activitas Nervosa Superior,* 1963, *5,* 373-390.

Bateson, G., Jackson, D.D., Haley, J., and Weakland, J. Toward a theory of schizophrenia. *Behavioral Science,* 1956, *1,* 251-264.

Becket, P.G.S., Senf, R., Frohman, C.E., and Gottlieb, S. Energy production and premorbid history in schizophrenia. *Archives of General Psychiatry,* 1963, *8*(2), 155-162.

213

Behrens, M., and Goldfarb, W. A study of patterns of interaction of families of schizophrenic children in residential treatment. *American Journal of Orthopsychiatry,* 1958, *28,* 300-312.

Bellak, L. A multiple-factor psychosomatic theory of schiozphrenia. *Psychiatric Quarterly,* 1949, *23,* 783.

Bellak, L. (Ed.). *Schizophrenic: A review of the syndrome.* New York: Logos, 1958.

Bender, L. Childhood schizophrenia. *Nervous Child,* 1942, *1,* 138.

Bender, L. Childhood schizophrenia: A clinical study of 100 schizophrenic children. *American Journal of Orthopsychiatry,* 1947(a), *17,* 40-56.

Bender, L. One hundred cases of child schizophrenics treated with shock. *Transactions American Neurological Association,* 1947(b), *72,* 161-169.

Bender, L. Childhood schizophrenia. *Psychiatric Quarterly,* 1953, *27,* 663-681.

Bender, L. *A dynamic psychopathology of childhood.* Springfield, Ill.: Charles C Thomas, 1954.

Bender, L. Schizophrenia in childhood—its recognition, description, and treatment. *American Journal of Orthopsychiatry,* 1956, *26,* 499-506.

Bender, L. The concept of pseudopsychopathic schizophrenia in adolescents. *American Journal of Orthopsychiatry,* 1959, *29,* 491-512.

Bender, L. Childhood schizophrenia. *International Journal of Psychiatry,* 1968, *5.*

Beres, D. Ego deviation and the concept of schizophrenia. *The Psychoanalytic Study of the Child,* 1956, *11,* 164-232.

Bergman, P., and Escalona, S.K. Unusual sensitivities in very young children. *The Psychoanalytic Study of the Child,* 1949, *3-4,* 333-352.

Bernfield, S. *The psychology of the infant.* London: Kegan, Paul, Trench, Trubner, & Co., Ltd., 1929.

Bettelheim, B. *Love is not enough.* Glencoe, Ill.: Free Press, 1950.

Bettelheim, B. *Truants from life; the rehabilitation of emotionally disturbed children.* Glencoe, Ill.: Free Press, 1955.

Bettelheim, B. Feral children and autistic children. *American Journal of Sociology,* 1959, *64,* 455-467.

Bettelheim, B. *The empty fortress: Infantile autism and the birth of self.* New York: Free Press, 1967.

Betz, B.J. A study of tactics for resolving the autistic barrier in the psychotherapy of the schizophrenic personality. *American Journal of Psychiatry,* 1947, *104,* 113-127.

Bishop, M.P. Effects of plasma from schizophrenic subjects upon learning and retention in the rat. In R.G. Heath (Ed.). *Serological fractions in schizophrenia.* New York: Harper & Row, 1963.

Bleuler, E. Autistic thinking. *American Journal of Insanity,* 1913, *69,* 873-886.

Bleuler, E. *Dementia praecox or the group of schizophrenias.* New York: International Universities Press, 1950.

Bleuler, M. *Endokrinologische Psychiatrie.* Stuttgart: Thieme, 1954.

Block, J., Patterson, V., Block, J., and Jackson, D. A study of the parents of schizophrenic and neurotic children. *Psychiatry*, 1958, *21*, 387-397.

Blos, P. *On adolescence*. Glencoe, Ill.: Free Press, 1962.

Boatman, M.J., and Szurek, S.A. A clinical study of childhood schizophrenia. In D.D. Jackson (Ed.). *The etiology of schizophrenia*. New York: Basic Books, 1960.

Böök, J.A. Genetical aspects of schizophrenic psychoses. In D.D. Jackson (Ed.). *The etiology of schizophrenia*. New York: Basic Books, 1960.

Bowen, M. A family concept in schizophrenia. In D.D. Jackson (Ed.). *The etiology of schizophrenia*. New York: Basic Books, 1960.

Bradley, C. Early evidence of psychoses in children with special reference to schizophrenia. *Journal of Pediatrics*, 1947, *30*, 529-540.

Brambilla, F., et al. Endocrinology in chronic schizophrenia. *Diseases of the Nervous System*, 1967, *28*(11), 745-748.

Brask, B.H. Borderline schizophrenia in children. *Acta Psychiatrica et Neurologica Scandinavia*, 1959, *34*, 265-282.

Brody, E.B., and Redlich, F.C. (Eds.). *Psychotherapy with schizophrenics: A symposium*. New York: International Universities Press, 1952.

Buck, C.W., Carscallan, H.B., and Hobbs, G.E. Temperature regulation in schizophrenia. *American Medical Association Archives in Neurology and Psychiatry*, 1950, *64*, 828-842.

Burstein, A.G. Some verbal aspects of primary process thought in schizophrenia. *Journal of Abnormal and Social Psychology*, 1961, *62*, 155-157.

Bychowski, G. *Psychotherapy of psychosis*. New York: Grune & Stratton, 1952.

Bykov, K. *The cerebral cortex and the inner organs*. New York: Chemical Publishing, 1957.

Call, J.D. Newborn approach behavior and early ego development. *International Journal of Psychoanalysis*, 1964, *45*, 286-295.

Cheek, F.E. The "schizophrenogenic mother" in word and deed. *Family Process*, 1964, *3*(1), 155-177.

Clardy, E.R., and Rumpf, E.M. The effect of electric shock treatment of children having schizophrenic manifestations. *Psychiatric Quarterly*, 1954, *28*, 616-623.

Clark, G. Reflection on the role of the mother in the development of language in the schizophrenic child. *Journal of the Canadian Psychiatric Association*, 1961, *6*, 252-256.

Colm, H. Phobias in children. *Psychoanalysis and Psychoanalytic Review*, 1959, *46*(3), 65-84.

Coolidge, J., Hahn, P.B., and Peck, A.L. School phobia, neurotic crises or way of life. *American Journal of Orthopsychiatry*, 1957, *27*, 296-309.

Cunningham, M.A. A five-year study of the language of an autistic child. *Journal of Child Psychology and Psychiatry*, 1966, *7*(2), 143-154.

Davidson, J.N. *The biochemistry of the nucleic acids*. New York: Wiley, 1960.

Davidson, S. School phobia as a manifestation of family disturbance: Its structure and treatment. *Journal of Child Psychology and Psychiatry*, 1961, *1*, 270-287.

Davis, D.R. The family triangle in schizophrenia. *British Journal of Medical Psychology*, 1961, *34*, 53-63.

DeMyer, M.K., Mann, N.A., Tilton, J.R., and Loew, L.H. Toy-play behavior and use of body by autistic and normal children as reported by mothers. *Psychological Reports*, 1967, *21*(3), 973-981.

Des Lauriers, A.M., and Halpern, F. Psychological tests in childhood schizophrenia. *American Journal of Orthopsychiatry*, 1947, *17*, 57-67.

Despert, J.L. Some considerations relating to the genesis of autistic behavior in children. *American Journal of Orthopsychiatry*, 1951, *21*, 335-350.

Despert, J.L. Diagnostic criteria of schizophrenia in children. *American Journal of Psychotherapy*, 1952, *6*, 148-163.

Despert, J.L. Differential diagnosis between obsessive-compulsive neurosis and schizophrenia in children. In P. Hoch and J. Zubin (Eds.). *Psychopathology of childhood*. New York: Grune & Stratton, 1955.

Despert, J.L., and Sherwin, A. Further examination of diagnostic criteria in schizophrenic illness and psychosis of infancy and early childhood. *American Journal of Psychiatry*, 1958, *114*, 784.

Deutsch, H. *Selected problems of adolescents*. New York: International Universities Press, 1967.

Doust, J. W. I. Spectroscopic and photoelectric oximetry in schizophrenia and other psychiatric states. *Journal of Mental Science*, 1952, *98*, 143-160.

Eickhoff, L. F. W. The aetiology of schizophrenia in childhood. *Journal of Mental Science*, 1952, *98*, 299-334.

Eisenberg, L. The autistic child in adolescence. *American Journal of Psychiatry*, 1956, *112*, 607-612.

Eisenberg, L. The course of childhood schizophrenia. *American Medical Association Archives of Neurology and Psychiatry*, 1957, *78*, 69-83.

Eisenson, J. *The psychology of speech*. New York: Appleton-Century Crofts, 1938.

Eissler, K. R. Remarks on the psychoanalysis of schizophrenia. In E.B. Brody and F.C. Redlich (Eds.) *Psychotherapy with schizophrenics: A symposium*. New York: International Universities Press, 1952.

Ekstein, R. Simultaneous treatment of a child and his mother. *American Journal of Psychotherapy*, 1953, *7*, 105-121.

Ekstein, R., and Wallerstein, J. Observations on the psychology of borderline and psychotic children. *The Psychoanalytic Study of the Child*, 1954, *9*, 344-369.

Ekstein, R., Friedman, S., and Caruth, E. The psychoanalytic treatment of childhood schizophrenia. In B.B. Wolman (Ed.). *Manual of child psychopathology*. New York: McGraw-Hill, 1970.

Erikson, E. *Identity: Youth and crisis*. New York: Norton, 1968.

Esman, A.H. Childhood psychosis and "childhood schizophrenia." *American Journal of Orthopsychiatry*, 1960, *30*, 391-396.

Esman, A., Kohn, M., and Nyman, L. The family of the schizophrenic child. *American Journal of Orthopsychiatry*, 1959, *29*, 455-459.

Farina, A. Patterns of role dominance and conflict in parents of schizophrenic patients. *Journal of Abnormal and Social Psychology,* 1960. *61,* 31-38.

Faris, R.E.L., and Dunham, H.W. *Mental disorders in urban areas.* Chicago: University of Chicago Press, 1939.

Federn, P. *Ego psychology and the psychoses.* New York: Basic Books, 1952.

Fenichel, O. *The psychoanalytic theory of neurosis.* New York: Norton, 1945.

Fish, B. Longitudinal observations of biological deviations in the schizophrenic infant. *American Journal of Psychiatry,* 1959, *116,* 25-31.

Fish, B. Involvement of the central nervous system of infants with schizophrenia. *Archives of Neurology,* 1960, *2,* 115-121.

Fleck, S., Lidz, T., Cornelison, A., Schafer, S., and Terry, D. The intrafamilial environment of the schizophrenic patient. In J.H. Masserman (Ed.). *Individual and family dynamics.* New York: Grune & Stratton, 1959.

Foudraine, J. Schizophrenia and the family: A survey of the literature 1956-1960 on the etiology of schizophrenia. *Acta Psychotherapeutica,* 1961, *9,* 82-110.

Fourbye, A., et al. Failure to detect 3,4-dimethoxyphenylethylamine in the urine of psychotic children. *Acta Psychiatrica Scandinavia,* 1966, *42,* Suppl. 191.

Freedman, A.M. Maturation and its relation to the dynamics of childhood schizophrenia. *American Journal of Orthopsychiatry,* 1954, *24,* 487-491.

Freedman, R. *Recent migration to Chicago.* Chicago: University of Chicago Press, 1950.

Freeman, H. Physiological studies. In L. Bellak, (Ed.). *Schizophrenia: A review of a syndrome.* New York: Logos, 1958.

Freud, A. Some remarks on infant observation. *The Psychoanalytic Study of the Child,* 1953, *8,* 9-19.

Freud, S. *Collected papers.* London: Hogarth Press and the Institute of Psychoanalysis, 1924-1950. 5 vols.

Freud, S. *The ego and the id.* London: Hogarth, 1927.

Friedhoff, A.J., and van Winkle, E. Isolation and characterization of a compound from the urine of schizophrenics. *Nature,* 1962, *194,* 897.

Gantt, W.H. *Physiological basis of psychiatry.* Springfield: Thomas, 1958.

Garcia, B., and Sarvis, M.A. Evaluation and treatment planning for autistic children. *Archives of General Psychiatry,* 1964, *10*(5), 530-541.

Garmezy, N. Stimulus differentiation of schizophrenic and normal subjects under conditions of reward and punishment. *Journal of Personality,* 1952, *20,* 253-276.

Garrone, G. Statistical genetic study of schizophrenia in the Geneva population between 1901-1950. *Journal of Genetics and Psychology,* 1962, 89-219.

Geleerd, E.R. A contribution to the problem of psychoses in childhood. *The Psychoanalytic Study of the Child,* 1946, *2,* 271-292.

Geleerd, E.R. The psychoanalysis of a psychotic child. *The Psychoanalytic Study of the Child,* 1949, *3-4,* 311-332.

Geleerd, E.R. Borderline states in childhood and adolescence. In J.W. Weinreb (Ed.). *Recent developments in psychoanalytic child therapy.* New York: International Universities Press, 1960.

Gerard, D.L., and Siegal, J. The family background of schizophrenia. *Psychiatric Quarterly*, 1950, *24*, 47-73.

German, G.A. Effects of serum from schizophrenic on evoked cortical potential in the rat. *British Journal of Psychiatry*, 1963, *109*, 616-623.

Gesell, A., and Amatruda, C.S. *Developmental diagnosis: Normal and abnormal child development: Clinical methods and pediatric applications* (2nd ed.). New York: Hoeber, 1947.

Gianascol, A. Psychodynamic approaches to childhood schizophrenia: A review. *Journal of Nervous and Mental Diseases*, 1963, *137*, 336-345.

Gittelman, M., and Birch, J.G. Childhood schizophrenia: Intellect, neurologic status, perinatal risk, prognosis and family pathology. *Archives of General Psychiatry*, 1967, *17*(1), 16-25.

Gjessing, R. Distribution of somatic function in catatonia with a periodic course and their compensation. *Journal of Mental Science*, 1938, *84*, 608.

Gjessing, L.R. Studies of periodic catatonia—I. Blood levels in protein-bound iodine and urinary excretion of vanillye-mandelic acid in relation to clinical course. *Journal of Psychiatric Research*, 1963, *2*, 123-124.

Goldberg, T.B. Factors in the development of school phobia. *Smith College Studies Social Work*, 1953, *23*, 227-248.

Goldfarb, W. Effects of psychological deprivation in infancy and subsequent stimulation. *American Journal of Psychiatry*, 1945 (a), *102*, 18-33.

Goldfarb, W. Psychological privation in infancy and subsequent adjustment. *American Journal of Orthopsychiatry*, 1945(b), *15*, 247-255.

Goldfarb, W. Receptor preferences in schizophrenic children. *American Medical Association Archives of Neurology and Psychiatry*, 1956, *76*, 643-653.

Goldfarb, W. Pain reactions in a groups of institutionalized schizophrenic children. *American Journal of Orthopsychiatry*, 1958, *28*, 777-785.

Goldfarb, W. *Childhood schizophrenia.* Cambridge: Harvard University Press, 1961.

Goldfarb, W., Braunstein, D., and Lorge, I. A study of speech patterns in a group of schizophrenic children. *American Journal of Orthopsychiatry.* 1956, *26*, 544-555.

Goldfarb, W., and Mintz, I. Schizophrenic child's reactions to time and space. *Archives of General Psychiatry*, 1961, *5*, 535-543.

Goldhamer, H., and Marshall, A.W. *Psychosis and civilization.* New York: Basic Books, 1949.

Goodenough, F.L. *Measurement of intelligence by drawing.* Tarrytown-on-Hudson, N.Y.: World, 1926.

Gottschalk, A. Further studies on the speech patterns of schizophrenic patients. *Journal of Nervous and Mental Diseases*, 1961, *132*, 101-113.

Gregory, I. Genetic factors in schizophrenia. *American Journal of Psychiatry*, 1960, *116*, 961-972.

Grosz, H., and Miller, I. Sibling patterns in schizophrenia. *Science*, 1958, *128*, 11-13.

Halpern, F. *A clinical approach to children's Rorschachs.* New York: Grune & Stratton, 1953.

Halpern, F. Diagnostic methods in childhood disorders. In B.B. Wolman (Ed.). *Handbook of clinical psychology.* New York: McGraw-Hill, 1965.

Hamburg, A.L. Orientation and defense reaction in simple and paranoid types of schizophrenia. In L.G. Voronin (Ed.). *The orientation reflex and orientating inquisitive behavior.* (Russ.) Moscow: Academia Pedagogicheskikh Nauk, 1958.

Hammer, E.F. *The clinical application of projective drawings.* Springfield, Ill.: Charles C Thomas, 1958.

Hare, E.H. Mental illness and social class in Bristol. *British Journal of Social Medicine,* 1955, *9,* 191-195.

Hartmann, J. Contribution to the metapsychology of schizophrenia. *The Psychoanalytic Study of the Child,* 1953, *8,* 177-198.

Heath, R.G. A. biochemical hypothesis on the etiology of schizophrenia. In D.D. Jackson (Ed.). *The etiology of schizophrenia.* New York: Basic Books, 1960.

Heath, R.G., and Krupp, I.M. Schizophrenia as a specific biologic disease. *American Journal of Psychiatry,* 1968, *124,* 1019-1027.

Hendrickson, W.J. Etiology in childhood schizophrenia. *Nervous Child,* 1952, *10,* 9-18.

Hill, L.B. *Psychotherapeutic intervention in schizophrenia.* Chicago: University of Chicago Press, 1955.

Hoagland, H. Metabolic and physiologic disturbances in the psychoses. In S. Cobb (Ed.). *The biology of mental health and disease.* New York: Hoeber, 1952.

Hollingshead, A.B., and Redlich, F.C. *Social class and mental illness.* New York: Wiley, 1958.

Hoskins, R.G. *The biology of schizophrenia.* New York: Norton, 1946.

Hurst, L. Etiology of mental disorders: Genetics. In B.B. Wolman (Ed.). *Manual of child psychopathology.* New York: McGraw-Hill, 1970.

Huston, P.E., and Shakow, D. Studies of motor function in schizophrenia. III. Steadiness. *Journal of Genetics and Psychology,* 1946, *34,* 119-126.

Hutt, C., and Ounsted, C. The biological significance of gaze aversion with particular reference to the syndrome of infantile autism. *Behavioral Science,* 1966, *11*(5), 346-356.

Hyden, H. Satellite cells in the nervous system. *Scientific American,* 1961, *205*(6), 62-70.

Ivanov-Smolensky, A.G. *Essays on the patho-physiology of higher nervous activity.* Moscow: Foreign Language Publishers, 1954.

Jackson, D.D. (Ed.). *The etiology of schizophrenia.* New York: Basic Books, 1960.

Jackson, D.D., and Weakland, J.H. Conjoint family therapy. *Psychiatry,* 1961, *24,* 30-45.

Johnson, A., Falstein, E.I., Szurck, S.A., and Svendsen, M. School phobia. *American Journal of Orthopsychiatry,* 1941, *9,* 702-711.

Kallmann, F.J. The genetic theory of schizophrenia. An analysis of 691 twin index families. *American Journal of Psychiatry,* 1946, *103,* 309-322.

Kallmann, F.J. *Heredity in health and mental disorder.* New York: Norton, 1953.

Kallmann, F.J. (Ed.). *Expanding goals of genetics in psychiatry.* New York: Grune & Stratton, 1962.

Kallmann, F.J., and Roth, B. Genetic aspects of preadolescent schizophrenia. *American Journal of Psychiatry,* 1956, *112,* 599-606.

Kanner, L. Autistic disturbances of affective contact. *Nervous Child,* 1943, *2,* 217-250.

Kanner, L. Early infantile autism. *Journal of Pediatrics,* 1944, *25,* 211-217.

Kanner, L. Irrelevant and metaphorical language in early infantile autism. *American Journal of Psychiatry,* 1946, *103,* 242-246.

Kanner, L. Problems of nosology and psychodynamics of early infantile autism. *American Journal of Orthopsychiatry,* 1949, *19,* 416-426.

Kanner, L. *Child psychiatry* (3rd ed.). Springfield, Ill.: Charles C Thomas, 1960.

Kanner, L., and Eisenberg, L. Notes on the follow-up studies of autistic children. In P.H. Hoch and J. Zubin (Eds.). *Psychopathology of childhood.* New York: Grune & Stratton, 1955.

Kanner, L., and Eisenberg, L. Early infantile autism, 1943-1955. *Psychiatric Research Reports,* 1957, (7), 55-66.

Karlsson, J.L. *The biologic basis of schizophrenia.* Springfield, Ill.: Charles C Thomas, 1966.

Kaufman, I., Thomas, F., Heims, L., Herrick, J., and Willer, L. Four types of defenses in mothers and fathers of schizophrenic children. *American Journal of Orthopsychiatry,* 1959, *29,* 460-472.

Kaufman, I., Thomas, F., Heims, L., Herrick, J., Reiser, D., and Willer, L. Treatment and implications of a new classification of parents of schizophrenic children. *American Journal of Psychiatry,* 1960, *116,* 920-924.

Kestenberg, J. Pseudo-schizophrenia in childhood and adolescence. *Nervous Child,* 1952, *10,* 146-163.

Kety, S.S. Recent biological theories of schizophrenia. In D.D. Jackson Ed.). *The etiology of schizophrenia.* New York: Basic Books, 1960.

Klebanoff, L. Parental attitudes of mothers of schizophrenic, brain injured, and retarded and normal children. *American Journal of Orthopsychiatry,* 1959, *29,* 445-454.

Klein, M. *Envy and gratitude.* New York: Basic Books, 1957.

Kline, N.S. Non-chemical factors and chemical theories of mental disease. In M. Rinkel and H.C.B. Denber (Eds.). *Chemical concepts of psychosis.* New York: McDowell, 1958.

Knight, R.P. Management and psychotherapy of the borderline schizophrenic patient. *Bulletin of the Menninger Clinic,* 1953, *17,* 139.

Kohn, M., and Clausen, J. Parental authority behavior and schizophrenia. *American Journal of Orthopsychiatry,* 1956, *26,* 297-313.

Kringlen, E. Discordance with respect to schizophrenia in monozygotic twins: Some genetic aspects. *Journal of Nervous and Mental Diseases,* 1964, *138,* 26-31.

Kringlen, E. Schizophrenia in twins: An epidemiological clinical study. *Psychiatry,* 1966, *29,* 172-184.

Kris, M. The use of prediction in a longitudinal study. *The Psychoanalytic Study of the Child,* 1957, *12,* 175-189.

Lemkau, P.V., and Crocetti, G.M. Vital statistics of schizophrenia. In L. Bellak (Ed.). *Schizophrenia: A review of the syndrome.* New York: Logos, 1958.

Leonberg, S.C., and Bok, J.B. Childhood schizophrenia: Organic or psychogenic? *Diseases of the Nervous System,* 1967, *28*(10), 686-687.

Lidz, T., Cornelison, A., Fleck, S., and Terry, D. The intrafamilial environment of schizophrenic patients: II. Marital schism and marital skew. *American Journal of Psychiatry,* 1957, *114,* 241-248.

Lidz, T., Cornelison, A., Terry, D., and Fleck, S. The intrafamilial environment of the schizophrenic patient: IV. Parental personalities and family interaction. *American Journal of Orthopsychiatry,* 1958, *28,* 764-776.

Lidz, T., and Fleck, S. Schizophrenia, human interaction and the role of the family. In D.D. Jackson (Ed.). *The etiology of schizophrenia.* New York: Basic Books, 1960.

Lidz, T., Schafer, S., Fleck, S., Cornelison, A., and Terry, D. Ego differentiation and schizophrenic symptom formation in identical twins. *Journal of the American Psychoanalytic Association,* 1962, *10,* 74-90.

Linton, R. *Culture and mental disorders.* Springfield, Ill.: Charles C Thomas, 1956.

Lu, Y.C. Mother-child role relations in schizophrenia. *Psychiatry,* 1961, *24,* 133-142.

Lu, Y.C. Contradictory parental expectations in schizophrenia. *Archives of General Psychiatry,* 1962, *6,* 219-234.

Lynn, R. Russian theory and research in schizophrenia. *Psychological Bulletin,* 1963, *60,* 486-498.

Machover, K. *Personality projection in the drawing of the human figure.* Springfield, Ill.: Charles C Thomas, 1949.

Mahler, M.S. Remarks on psychoanalysis with psychotic children. *Quarterly Journal of Child Behavior,* 1949, *1,* 18-21.

Mahler, M.S. On child psychosis and schizophrenia. Autistic and symbiotic infantile phychoses. *The Psychoanalytic Study of the Child,* 1952, *7,* 286-305.

Mahler, M.S. Discussion of Chaps. 13-16. In P. Hoch et al. (Eds.). *Psychopathology of childhood.* New York: Grune & Stratton, 1955.

Mahler, M.S. Autism and symbiosis, two extreme disturbances of identity. *International Journal of Psychoanalysis,* 1958, *39,* 1-7.

Mahler, M.S. On sadness and grief in infancy and childhood: Loss and restoration of the symbiotic love object. *The Psychoanalytic Study of the Child,* 1961, *16,* 332-351.

Mahler, M.S. *On human symbiosis and the vicissitudes of individuation.* New York: International Universities Press, 1968.

Mahler, M.S., and Elkisch, P. Some observations on disturbances of the ego in a case of infantile psychosis. *The Psychoanalytic Study of the Child,* 1953, *8,* 252-261.

Mahler, M.S., and Gosliner, B.J. On symbiotic child psychosis: Genetic, dynamic and restitutive aspects. *The Psychoanalytic Study of the Child,* 1955, *10,* 195-214.

Malis, G.A. *Research on the etiology of schizophrenia.* New York: Consultants Bureau, 1961.

Malzberg, B., and Lee, E.S. *Migration and mental disease.* New York: Social Science Research Council, 1956.

McCarthy, D. Research in language development: Retrospect and prospect. *Monographs of the Society for Research in Child Development,* 1959, *24*(5), 3-24.

Mednick, S.A. A learning theory approach to research in schizophrenia. *Psychological Bulletin,* 1958, *55,* 316-327.

Mehr, H.M, The application of psychological tests and methods to schizophrenia in children. *Nervous Child,* 1952, *10,* 63-93.

Merton, R., and Kendall, P.L. The focused interview. *American Journal of Sociology,* 1964, *51,* 541-557.

Michaux, L., and Dugas, M. La névrose obsessionelle chez l'enfant. *Presse Thermale Clinique,* 1959, *96*(1), 5-12.

Midelfort, C.F. *The family in psychotherapy.* New York: McGraw-Hill, 1957.

Milt, H. Serious mental illness in children. *Public Affairs,* 1963, *352.*

Money, J., and Hirsch, S.R. Chromosome anomalies, mental deficiency and schizophrenia. *Archives of General Psychiatry,* 1963, *8,* 242-251.

Morris, J.V. Cases of elective mutism. *American Journal of Mental Deficiency,* 1953, *57,* 661-668.

Nagelberg, L., Spotnitz, H., and Feldman, Y. An attempt at healthy insulation in the withdrawn child. *American Journal of Orthopsychiatry,* 1953, *13,* 238-252.

Neubauer, P., and Steinhert, J. Schizophrenia in adolescence. *Nervous Child,* 1952, *10,* 129-134.

Norman, E. Reality relationships of schizophrenic children. *British Journal of Medicine and Psychology,* 1954, *27,* 126-141.

Norman, E. Affect and withdrawal in schizophrenic children. *British Journal of Medicine and Psychology,* 1955, *28,* 1-18.

Nuffield, E.J.A. The schizogenic mother. *Medical Journal of Australia,* 1954, *2,* 283-286.

Ødegaard, O. Emigration and insanity. *Acta Psychiatrica et Neurologica,* 1932, *4.*

Ødegaard, O. The distribution of mental diseases in Norway. *Acta Psychiatrica et Neurologica,* 1945, *20,* 247-284.

Ornitz, E.M., and Ritvo, E.R. Perceptual inconsistency in early infantile autism. *Archives of General Psychiatry,* 1968, *18*(1), 76-98.

Osmond, H., and Hoffer, A. A comprehensive theory of schizophrenia. *International Journal of Neuropsychiatry,* 1966, *2,* 302-309.

Overholser, W., and Werkman, S. Etiology, pathogenesis, and pathology. In L. Bellak (Ed.). *Schizophrenia: A review of the syndrome.* New York: Logos, 1958.

Owen, M. Over-identification in the schizophrenic child and its relationship to treatment. *Journal of Nervous and Mental Diseases,* 1955, *121,* 223-229.

Pasamanick, B., and Knoblock, H. Early feeding and birth difficulties in childhood schizophrenia: An exploratory note. *Journal of Psychology,* 1963, *56*(1), 73-77.

Pascal, G.R., Swenson, C.H., et al. Prognostic criteria in the case histories of hospitalized mental patients. *Journal of Consultant Psychology,* 1953, *17,* 163-171.

Pavlov, I.P. *Lectures on conditioned reflexes.* New York: Liveright, 1928.

Peck, H. Rabinovitch, R., and Cramer, J. A treatment program for parents of schizophrenic children. *American Journal of Orthopsychiatry* 1949, *19,* 592-598.

Piotrowski, Z.A. A comparison of congenitally defective children with schizophrenic children in regard to personality structure and intelligence type. *Proceedings of the American Association of Mental Deficiencies,* 1937, *42,* 78-90.

Piotrowski, Z.A. Experimental psychological diagnosis of mild forms of schizophrenia. *Rorschach Research Exchange,* 1945, *9,* 189-200.

Planansky, K. Heredity in schizophrenia. *Journal of Nervous and Mental Diseases,* 1955, *122,* 121-142.

Pollin, W., Stabenau, J.R., and Tupin, J. Family studies with identical twins discordant for schizophrenia. *Psychiatry,* 1965, *28,* 60-78.

Pronovost, P. Speech behavior and language comprehension of autistic children. *Journal of Chronic Diseases,* 1961, *13,* 228-233.

Putnam, M.C. Some observations on psychosis in early childhood. In G. Caplan (Ed.). *Emotional problems of early childhood.* New York: Basic Books, 1955.

Rabin, A., and Haworth, M. *Projective techniques with children.* New York: Grune & Stratton, 1960.

Rachman, S., and Costello, C.G. The aetiology and treatment of children's phobias: A review. *American Journal of Psychiatry,* 1961, *118,* 97-105.

Rank, B. Adaption of the psychoanalytic technique for the treatment of young children with atypical development. *American Journal of Orthopsychiatry,* 1949, *19,* 130-139.

Rank, B. Intensive study of preschool children who show marked personality deviations or "atypical development" and their parents. In G. Caplan (Ed.). *Emotional problems of early childhood.* New York: Basic Books, 1955.

Redl, F. and Wineman, D. *Children who hate* (2nd ed.). New York: Free Press, 1960.

Reiss, M. Correlations between changes in mental states and thyroid activity after different forms of treatment. *Journal of Mental Science,* 1954, *100,* 687-703.

224   REFERENCES

Ribble, M.A., Redl, F., and Wineman, D. Clinical studies of instinctive reactions in newborn babies. *American Journal of Psychiatry, 1938, 15.*

Richards, B.W. Childhood schizophrenics and mental deficiency. *Journal of Mental Science, 1951, 97, 290-372.*

Richter, D. (Ed.). *Schizophrenia: Somatic aspects.* New York: Macmillan, 1957.

Rimland, B. *Infantile autism.* New York: Appleton-Century -Crofts, 1964.

Robinson, F. The psychoses of early childhood. *American Journal of Orthopsychiatry, 1961, 31, 536-550.*

Rosen, J.N. *Direct analysis.* New York: Grune & Stratton, 1953.

Rosenthal, D. Some factors associated with concordance and discordance with respect to schizophrenia in monozygotic twins. *Journal of Nervous and Mental Diseases, 1959, 129, 1-10.*

Rosenthal, D. Confusion of identity and the frequency of schizophrenia in twins. *Archives of General Psychiatry, 1960, 3, 297-304.*

Rosenthal, D. Problems of sampling and diagnosis in the major twin studies of schizophrenia. *Journal of Psychiatric Research, 1962, 1, 116-134.*

Rosenthal, D. The offspring of schizophrenic couples. *Journal of Psychiatric Research, 1966, 4, 169-188.*

Roth, M. Interaction of genetic and environmental factors in the causation of schizophrenia. In D. Richter (Ed.). *Schizophrenia: Somatic aspects.* New York: Macmillan, 1957.

Sabbath, J.C. Infantilization of a preschool child. In G. Caplan (Ed.). *Emotional problems of early childhood.* New York: Basic Books, 1955.

Sackler, M.D., Sackler, R.R., LaBurt, H.A., Tui, C., and Sackler, A.M. A psychobiologic viewpoint of schizophrenia in childhood. *Nervous Child, 1952, 10, 43-59.*

Sands, D.E. The psychoses of adolescence. *Journal of Mental Science, 1956, 102, 308-318.*

Sanua, V.D. Sociocultural factors in families of schizophrenics: A review of literature. *Psychiatry, 1961, 24, 246-265.*

Schacter, F., Meyer, L., and Loomis, E. Childhood schizophrenia and mental retardation: Differential diagnosis before and after one year of psychotherapy. *American Journal of Orthopsychiatry, 1962, 32, 584-595.*

Schmidelberg, M. A note on obsessional indecision. *Psychoanalytic Review, 1948, 35, 312-313.*

Schneidman, E.S. The MAPS Test with children. In A. Rabin and M. Haworth (Eds.). *Projective techniques with children.* New York: Grune & Stratton, 1960, 130-148.

Schulman, I. Concept formation in the schizophrenic child: A study of ego development. *Journal of Clinical Psychology, 1953, 9, 11-15.*

Shapiro, D. Aspects of obsessive-compulsive style. *Psychiatry, 1962, 25(1), 46-59.*

Sherman, M., and Beverly, B.J. Hallucinations in children, *Journal of Abnormal and Social Psychology, 1924, 19, 165.*

Shulgin, A.T., et al. Role of 3,4-dimethoxyphenyl-ethylamine in schizophrenia and other conditions. *Nature, 1967, 214, 484-485.*

Slater, E. Psychotic and neurotic illnesses in twins. *Medical Research Council, Special Report 278.* London: His Majesty's Stationery Office, 1953.

Slater, E. The monogenic theory of schizophrenia. *Acta Genetica,* 1958, *8,* 50-56.

Soble, D. Some observations of childhood schizophrenia. *Psychiatric Quarterly Supplement,* 1955, *29,* 272-280.

Sontag, L.W. The possible relationship of prenatal environment to schizophrenia. In D.D. Jackson (Ed.). *The etiology of schizophrenia.* New York: Basic Books, 1960.

Sorosky, A., Ornitz, E.M., Brown, M.B., and Ritvo, E.R. Systematic observations of autistic behavior. *Archives of General Psychiatry,* 1968, *18,* 439-450.

Spitz, R.A. Hospitalism—an inquiry into the genesis of psychiatric conditions in early childhood. *The Psychoanalytic Study of the Child,* 1945, *1,* 53-74.

Spitz, R.A. Anaclitic depression, an inquiry into the genesis of psychiatric conditions in early childhood. *The Psychoanalytic Study of the Child,* 1946a, *2,* 313-342.

Spitz, R.A. Hospitalism: A follow-up report. *The Psychoanalytic Study of the Child,* 1946b, *2,* 113-117.

Spitz, R.A. *The first year of life.* New York: International Universities Press, 1965.

Sullivan, H.S. *Conceptions of modern psychiatry.* Washington, D.C.: W.A. White, 1947.

Sullivan, H.S. *The interpersonal theory of psychiatry.* New York: Norton, 1953.

Sullivan, H.S. *Schizophrenia as a human process.* New York: Norton, 1962.

Symonds, A., and Herman, M. The patterns of schizophrenia in adolescence. *Psychiatric Quarterly,* 1957, *31,* 521-530.

Szára, S. The comparison of the psychotic effect of tryptamine derivatives with the effects of mescaline and LSD-25 in self experiments. In S. Garattini and V. Ghetti (Eds.). *Psychotropic drugs.* London: Cleaver-Hume Press, 1958.

Szurek, S.A. Psychotic episodes and psychotic maldevelopment. *American Journal of Orthopsychiatry,* 1956, *26,* 519-543.

Taft, L.T., and Goldfarb, W. Prenatal and perinatal factors in childhood schizophrenia. *Developmental Medicine and Child Neurology,* 1964, *6*(1), 32-43.

Talbot, M. Panic in school phobia. *American Journal of Orthopsychiatry,* 1957, *27,* 286-295.

Tec, L. A schizophrenic child becomes adolescent. *Journal of Nervous and Mental Diseases,* 1955, *122,* 105.

Thomes, M.M. Parents of schizophrenic and normal children: A comparison of parental attitudes and marital adjustment, role behavior, and interaction. *Dissertation Abstract,* 1959, *20,* 2413.

Tilton, J.F., and Ottinger, D.R. Comparison of the toy play behavior of autistic, retarded, and normal children. *Psychological Reports*, 1964, *15*, 967-975.

Toolan, J.M. Suicide and suicidal attempts in children and adolescents. *American Journal of Psychiatry*, 1962, *118*, 719-724.

Von Brauchitsch, H.K., and Kirk, W.E. Childhood schizophrenia and social class. *American Journal of Orthopsychiatry*, 1967, *37*(2), 400.

Von Studnitz, N. Excretion of 3,4-dimethoxyphenyl-ethlamine in schizophrenia. *Acta Psychiatrica Scandinavia*, 1965, *41*, 117-121.

Vorster, D. An investigation into the part played by organic factors in childhood schizophrenia. *Journal of Mental Science*, 1960, *106*, 494-522.

Walaszek, E.J. Brain neurohormones and cortical epinephrine pressor responses as affected by schizophrenic serum. *International Review of Neurobiology*, 1960, *2*, 137.

Waldfogel, S., Coolidge, J., and Hahn, P. The development, meaning and management of school phobia. *American Journal of Orthopsychiatry*, 1957, *27*, 754-780.

Wallinga, J. Separation anxiety-school phobia. *Journal Lancet*, 1959, *79*, 258-260.

Waring, M., and Ricks, D. Family patterns of children who became adult schizophrenics. *Journal of Nervous and Mental Diseases*, 1965, *140*(5), 351-364.

Weakland, J.H. The double-bind hypothesis of schizophrenia and three party interaction. In D.D. Jackson (Ed.). *The etiology and schizophrenia*. New York: Basic Books, 1960.

Wechsler, D., and Jaros, E. Schizophrenic patterns on the WISC. *Journal of Clinical Psychology*, 1965, *21*, 288-291.

Weil, A. Clinical data and dynamic considerations in certain cases of childhood schizophrenia. *American Journal of Orthopsychiatry*, 1953, *23*, 518-529.

Weinberg, S.K. Social psychological aspects of schizophrenia. In L. Appleby, J.M. Scher, and J. Cumming (Eds.). *Chronic schizophrenia*. Glencoe, Ill.: The Free Press, 1960, 68-85.

Werkman, S.L. Present trends in schizophrenia research: Implications for childhood schizophrenia. *American Journal of Orthopsychiatry*, 1959, *29*, 473-480.

Wexler, M. The structural problem in schizophrenia. In M. Brody and F. C. Redlich (Eds.). *Psychotherapy with schizophrenics*. New York: International Universities Press, 1952.

Whitaker, C.A. (Ed.). *Psychotherapy of chronic schizophrenic patients*. Boston: Little, Brown, 1958.

Whitehorn, J.C. Psychodynamic approach to the study of psychosis. In F. Alexander and N. Ross (Eds.). *Dynamic psychiatry*. Chicago: University Press, 1952.

Williams, C.H., et al. 3,4-dimethoxyphenyl-ethylamine in schizophrenia. *Nature*, 1966, *211*, 1195.

Winder, C.L. Some psychological studies of schizophrenis. In D.D. Jackson (Ed.). *The etiology of schizophrenia.* New York: Basic Books, 1960.

Wittenborn, J.R. Depression. In B.B. Wolman (Ed.). *Handbook of clinical psychology.* New York: McGraw-Hill, 1965.

Wittman, M., and Huffman, A. A comparative study of the developmental adjustment and personality characteristics of psychotic, psychoneurotic delinquent and normally adjusted teen-age youth. *Journal of General Psychology,* 1945, *66,* 167-182.

Wolman, B.B. *The neurasthenic child.* (Polish) 1933.

Wolman, B.B. Mentally disturbed children. (Hebrew) In I. Rivkai (Ed.). *The handbook of mother and child.* Tel Aviv: Sick Rund, 1936.

Wolman, B.B. Diagnosis in clinical psychology. (Hebrew.) *Hed Hachinuch,* 1943, *18,* 17-21.

Wolman, B.B. Juvenile delinquents in Palestine. (Hebrew.) *Hachinuch Quarterly,* 1946, *17,* 50-79.

Wolman, B.B. Intellectual development in adolescence. (Hebrew.) *Hachinuch Quarterly,* 1948, *19,* 131-148.

Wolman, B.B. Disturbances in acculturation. *American Journal of Psychotherapy,* 1949, *3,* 601-615.

Wolman, B.B. The Jewish adolescent. *Jewish Social Studies,* 1951, *13,* 333-344.

Wolman, B.B. Leadership and group dynamics. *Journal of Social Psychology,* 1956, *43,* 11-25.

Wolman, B.B. Explorations in latent schizophrenia. *American Journal of Psychotherapy,* 1957, *11,* 560-588.

Wolman, B.B. Instrumental, mutual acceptance, and vectorial groups. *Acta Sociologica,* 1958(a), *3,* 19-28.

Wolman, B.B. The deterioration of the ego in schizophrenia. Paper presented at *Eastern Psychological Association,* 1958(b).

Wolman, B.B. Impact of failure on group cohesiveness. *Journal of Social Psychology,* 1960, *51,* 409-418.

Wolman, B.B. The fathers of schizophrenic patients. *Acta Psychotherapeutica,* 1961, *9,* 193-210.

Wolman, B.B. Non-participant observation on a closed ward. *Acta Psychotherapeutica,* 1964, *12,* 61-71.

Wolman, B.B. Family dynamics and schizophrenia. *Journal of Health and Human Behavior,* 1965(a).

Wolman, B.B. Mental health and mental disorders. In B.B. Wolman (Ed.). *Handbook of clinical psychology.* New York: McGraw-Hill, 1965(b).

Wolman, B.B. Schizophrenia and related disorders. In B.B. Wolman (Ed.). *Handbook of clinical psychology.* New York: McGraw-Hill, 1965(c).

Wolman, B.B. *Vectoriasis praecox or the group of schizophrenias.* Springfield, Ill.: Charles C Thomas, 1966.

Wolman, B.B. The socio-psycho-somatic theory of schizophrenia. *Psychotherapy and Psychosomatics,* 1967, *15,* 373-387.

Wolman, B.B. *Call no man normal.* New York: 1970(a).

Wolman, B.B. *Adolescents in a changing society.* New York: Free Press, 1970(b).

Wolpe, J., and Rachman, S. Psychoanalytic "evidence": A critique based on Freud's case of little Hans. *Journal of Nervous and Mental Diseases,* 1960, *131*, 135-148.

Wooley, D.W. Serotonin in mental disorders. *Research Publications of the Association for Nervous and Mental Diseases,* 1958, *36*, 381-400.

Wynne, L.C., and Rychoff, I.M. Pseudo-mutuality in the family relations in schizophrenics. *Psychiatry,* 1958, *21*, 205-220.

Author Index

Subject Index

Date Due

APR 8 '74			
NOV 1 3 74			
APR. 1 3 1976			
OCT 8 1980			
OCT 2 8 1980			
FEB 1 6 1982			
FEB 2 2 1983			
APR 1 4 1983			
OCT 2 8 1983			
JAN 6 1984	MA 8 '90		
FEB 11 1984	JA 29 '90		
MAY 4 1986	FE 20 '90		
OC 8 '85	NO 2 4 08		
OC 1 6 '87			
NO 6 '87			
NO 10 '89			

Demco 38-297